Praise for *Eat [...]*

"Dawn Harris Sherling distills food history in the United States and food science to an actionable plan for healthy living. With delicious, anti-inflammatory recipes, this is the perfect companion for anyone struggling with IBS, type 2 diabetes, weight control, and other digestive disorders."

—**Dan Buettner, National Geographic Fellow and
#1** *New York Times* **bestselling author of** *The Blue Zones*

"The author has years of experience and in-depth knowledge of both the good and the bad of the foods we eat. She shares her passion for good food and good health in an engaging book that should be on everyone's shelf."

—**Stuart Mushlin, MD, MACP, master clinician
in internal medicine and primary care and author of**
Playing the Ponies and Other Medical Mysteries Solved

"*Eat Everything* by Dawn Harris Sherling, MD, is a must-read for anyone with a digestive disorder, diabetes, or difficulty with weight loss. In lucid terms, Dr. Sherling describes the beneficial elements of whole foods and the hazards of additives using state of the art information and medical experience which will improve your health and well-being."

—**Lester Rosen, MD, former president of the
American Society of Colon and Rectal Surgeons**

"Dawn Harris Sherling is a relatable, reliable guide when it comes to understanding the importance of digestive well-being, and the dangers of food additives and ultra-processed foods. Listen to her advice, take care of yourself, and learn how to *Eat Everything*!"

—**Kathryn M. Rexrode, MD, MPH, chief of the division
of women's health at Brigham and Women's Hospital and
professor of medicine at Harvard Medical School**

"Dr. Sherling presents a clear, practical, and sustainable approach to eating that may relieve gastrointestinal symptoms and improve overall health."

—**Spencer Dorn, MD, MPH, MHA, vice chair and professor of
medicine at the University of North Carolina and gastroenterologist**

Eat Everything

Also by Dawn Harris Sherling

Not Quite Dead: a Novel

Eat

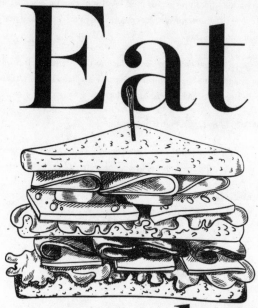

Everything

How to **Ditch** Additives and Emulsifiers, **Heal** Your Body, and **Reclaim** the Joy of Food

Dawn Harris Sherling, MD

BenBella Books, Inc.
Dallas, TX

Eat Everything copyright © 2023 by Dawn Harris Sherling

BenBella Books, Inc.
10440 N. Central Expressway
Suite 800
Dallas, TX 75231
benbellabooks.com
Send feedback to feedback@benbellabooks.com

BenBella is a federally registered trademark.

Printed in the United States of America
10 9 8 7 6 5 4 3 2 1

Library of Congress Control Number: 2022045485
ISBN 9781637742594 (trade paperback)
ISBN 9781637742600 (electronic)

Editing by Claire Schulz
Copyediting by Ruth Strother
Proofreading by Cape Cod Compositors and W. Brock Foreman
Indexing by WordCo Indexing Services
Text design and composition by Sarah Avinger
Cover design by Faceout Studio, Molly von Borstel
Cover photography © Adobe Stock / fahrwasser and © Shutterstock / Ton Photographer 4289
Photo by Sally Prissert, W Studio
Interior illustrations © Adobe Stock / Aleksey (Sandwich with Toothpick), vectorgoods (Spoon, Bread Grouping, and Cheese Carving), Kate Macate (Vegetable Grouping, Supermarket Basket, and Dairy Grouping), and jenesesimre (Pizza)
Printed by Lake Book Manufacturing

Special discounts for bulk sales are available. Please contact bulkorders@benbellabooks.com.

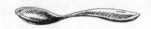

For Michael, Eli, and Julia.

Ess gezunterheit.

Author's Note

This book is based on research, interviews with leading experts, and my experiences as a physician and as a patient. In this book, patients' names have been changed, and in some cases their stories have been combined to protect their anonymity.

Contents

Part III: Eating Everything in Real Life

Introduction

Emma is a patient I will never forget. That's because doctors forever remember the patients we failed.

Emma, a bespectacled twenty-three-year-old accompanied by her mother, came to me not for a second opinion but for what must have seemed like a last chance long shot. She had driven down to Boston from Maine, which was my first clue that something was really wrong. Mainers are the toughest of New Englanders and make that hours-long drive for medical care only when they are in dire straits. By the time she showed up to see me at the Brigham and Women's Hospital outpatient office where I worked, Emma was subsisting mostly on granola bars. She said that if she tried to eat anything else, she would spend the day with a bloated belly and nauseated, and she would have to run to the toilet to evacuate her bowels but never feel as if she had experienced a complete bowel movement. Sticking to the granola bars helped her, but she still felt slightly nauseous all the time.

She had been evaluated by a gastroenterologist (a specialist that focuses on the stomach and intestines), who tested Emma for celiac disease and had done several additional tests, including an upper endoscopy and colonoscopy to rule out the possibility of other diseases. She had also seen an infectious disease specialist, an endocrinologist, a dietician, and a psychiatrist. None of the medications she had tried provided her with much relief. She had been told she had anxiety, an eating disorder, and irritable bowel syndrome (IBS). Despite her best efforts at incorporating dietary advice from the dietician, this hadn't helped her much either.

As I reviewed Emma's records, I realized I didn't have much else to offer her. Her workup had been pretty thorough. But Emma's mother insisted it was not "all in her head" as her doctors in Maine had ultimately decided. Her mother knew Emma as only a parent can know her child and was convinced something was physically wrong with her. Her formerly happy, productive daughter had become miserable and was afraid to eat and go out.

I had recently finished my primary care internal medicine residency at the Brigham after graduating cum laude from the Yale School of Medicine and was now an Instructor of Medicine at Harvard University. I thought I knew a lot. But from working at one of the best medical centers in the country, I understood there were people who were much smarter and more experienced than I was. So I referred Emma to them. She saw another gastroenterologist and endocrinologist. She had more tests—all showing no evidence of physical disease. And then she came back to see me.

Without a blood test, biopsy, or scan specifically designed to diagnose it, IBS is known as a diagnosis of exclusion, meaning other diseases are searched for, and if they aren't found and it sounds like the person has IBS, that's the diagnosis they are given. Since so few treatments are available for IBS and there is thought to be a powerful brain-gut connection, I suggested that a psychologist in Maine might be her best bet. She agreed to find a psychologist on her own, and both she and her mother stood up, shoulders heavy, eyes cast down, and left my office for the last time.

Shortly thereafter, as a new mom tired of Boston's unforgiving winters and with a lack of extended family in the area, I decided to return to my home state of Florida. I didn't see Emma again, but I could never shake the feeling that something else *had* been going on with her, something that I couldn't quite figure out at the time. Emma was the first patient I had seen who was able to clearly articulate that what she was eating had an obvious effect on her health, but she certainly wasn't the last one to tell me that. The problem was that neither Emma nor anyone else could sort out what it was that was making her feel so ill.

Years passed, and though not as severely as Emma, I started to feel ill after eating, too. I began to develop IBS, and it was getting worse.

I first decided to cut out dairy, proclaiming myself lactose intolerant. When that didn't help much, after about six months, I got rid of bread and other foods containing gluten. A year later, becoming increasingly frustrated, I started on a low-FODMAP diet—short for low in fermentable oligosaccharides, disaccharides, monosaccharides, and polyols (more on this in chapter 1)—the highly restrictive eating plan that had become the medical standard for patients with IBS. The list of foods I was supposed to avoid was long. Patients to whom I had recommended low-FODMAP would come back from the dietician and plead, "Just tell me what I *can* eat!" Like my patients, I hated the low-FODMAP diet. It made me feel as though I couldn't enjoy normal life. The science behind it is solid, but the commitment to it was challenging to the point of being near impossible to stick with—and it doesn't work as well as most patients need it to. Ultimately, many IBS sufferers give it up, but I had been led to believe that food avoidance was the best treatment there was.

After a year, I was mentally and physically exhausted from trying to get my bowels to behave. But I was determined not to let my IBS get in the way of family activities, especially not when my husband and I decided to plan a trip to Italy with the kids. Everyone was excited for our vacation, including me. Although privately I wondered if I would be able to enjoy the food in Italy at all. Bread, garlic, onions, cheese—all these critical components of Italian cuisine were on my avoid list. Traveling to Italy was a tremendous privilege, and I vowed I would figure it out.

———————————————

On the road to Rome, the over-airconditioned tour bus eased its way into the highway rest stop parking lot, pulling up next to the nondescript yellow stucco building distinguished only by its bright-red roof. Our jet-lagged group trudged off the bus in a line toward the combination quick-serve restaurant and convenience store. But for the Italian words on the sign, this could have been a rest stop nearly anywhere in the US.

My first real Italian meal was at a place called the Autogrill. The unappetizing name notwithstanding, our tour guides assured us that the food would be good here. We were told to order our pasta dish at one side, pay for it, and present the receipt to the food servers. If we wanted coffee, it would have to be ordered separately at the far side of the establishment. Rest stop pasta was not exactly the culinary experience I was hoping to have in Italy. I took my place in line, envisioning oily noodles covered by a heavily salted, runny sauce, sitting in chafing dishes.

But despite my initial impression, this rest stop in Italy was not at all the same as a rest stop in the US. Within a few minutes I realized there were no chafing dishes, and the only oil I saw was the small amount put into the pan as one cook heated the fresh marinara sauce I had ordered while another dipped the pasta into boiling water. When al dente perfection had been reached, she brought the drained pasta over to the pan and neatly added it to the marinara, deftly turning it to coat every (dangerously gluten-filled) strand with the (perilously acidic) red sauce. Freshly grated cheese was added (oh no!), and I was then handed an honest-to-goodness ceramic dinner plate. Small puffs of steam wafted from the dish, the garlicky aroma making me a little giddy. To think this was what passed for fast food in Italy! I pushed aside my fears and decided that I was going to enjoy my trip—which meant this would be lunch. I couldn't help but eat every bite, only vaguely wondering how much garlic and onion might be in the sauce.

Whatever the consequences of my meal, surely the fresh pasta would be worth the bathroom drama that might later ensue (in any case, the journey to our hotel was expected to be short). And yet the bus ride turned out to be blissfully uneventful, save my children squabbling about something or other. To my surprise, I didn't feel heavy or bloated after my large plate of spaghetti. Actually, I felt great—newly energized for our Italian adventure.

Despite this success, I reminded myself to be cautious. Over the last several years, my bowels had become unpredictable. Like Emma, I hadn't been able to figure out any pattern, but my problem was clearly linked to what I was eating. Some days were terrible, with everything I ate struggling to find its way through my intestinal twists and turns, and some days I hardly noticed my gut at all. On my first day in Italy, the gods of intestines must have been smiling down on me—perhaps I would be okay that day but suffer on another. So later that evening, I decided I would try only small bites of my kids' gelato and wait for the inevitable disaster.

Hours passed. Then a whole day. Nothing happened. I bravely decided to move on to my own gelato. Another uneventful day, so then I began requesting the fresh whipped cream on top, too. And still, my bowels were behaving. Within three days of being in Italy, we had consumed an embarrassingly large amount of gelato. (In our defense, the weather was very warm.) And not only had nothing bad happened, but somehow, without trying, my bowels were back to normal—like when I was a medical resident in my twenties downing pepper and onion pizza. I ecstatically feasted my way through the country, eating everything from creamy *cacio e pepe* pasta in Rome to giant cuts of steak in Florence to inexplicably light, crusty, and doughy Neapolitan pizza topped with fresh *mozzarella di bufala* wherever it was offered. I wasn't thinking about my intestines at all. It was a great trip.

Sadly, the day after returning to the US, my bowels were back to misbehaving. What was different in Italy? Had it been the walking? The lowered stress of being on vacation? Maybe I had been eating more roughage (the fruits and veggies had been delicious, after all). I was disappointed and tried to walk more, eat more fiber but to no avail. My IBS was back in full force.

And then, amazingly, we were able to go back to Italy the following summer. I didn't know what would happen, but this time I didn't hesitate to begin my eating adventure. And again, within a day, my bowels had normalized. This trip, however, there was less walking and more stress, eliminating lack of exercise and higher emotional distress as causes of my IBS. It most definitely wasn't in my head, and it wasn't in my legs, either. And then I remembered my patients who had gone on whole-food diets telling me their IBS had gotten better, and I started to wonder what was in the Italian food that wasn't in my food back home? Or perhaps was it the other way around?

Italians take a great deal of pride in preparing their food, and eating is a source of joy, not discomfort or restriction. Where we visited, chefs had not yet given up on scratch cooking (if something wasn't fresh, it was noted on the menu). They used fresh, in-season ingredients and, more so than Americans, avoided ultra-processed substitutes. Italians also don't suffer from IBS, diabetes, or obesity at the rates Americans do. Could these things possibly be related? Both for my own health and that of my patients, I decided I'd make it my mission to find out.

What I began to realize in Italy, and by paying closer attention to my patients, eventually became an investigation that turned everything I thought I knew about what we should be eating on its head. This book is a culmination of those efforts. I discovered that IBS is just the canary in a coal mine of a host of diet-related diseases like fatty liver and diabetes. Although I first attributed my IBS cure to something amorphous in the Italian ether, the truth was that the ingredients I was eating there were whole and simple—most importantly, free of the additives (artificial sweeteners, emulsifiers, and thickeners) that have become ubiquitous in most Americans' diets.

To be clear, I'm not just talking about the junk food and greasy drive-through fare that many of us picture when we hear the familiar lament about the standard American diet. As with many of my patients, I thought I was eating healthfully—I shunned fast food, ate salads often, and filled my shopping cart with packages promising the contents were sugar-free or plant-based or whole or natural. And yet I was spending an hour a day on the toilet, and I was miserable.

So I began reading. Every day I scanned my food packages and found a new ingredient to look up. To my surprise, there was evidence that many of the additives I was eating had significant effects on the microbiome (the bacteria, fungi, and viruses that live in our intestines), which we are learning can have wide-ranging effects not only on our gastrointestinal system, but on how much we weigh, our moods, and even our immune system. The evidence I found wasn't on some fringe website but in highly respected peer-reviewed journals like *Nature, Cell, Gut,* and *Gastroenterology*.

Then, as I was working on this manuscript, societies like the International Organization for the Study of Inflammatory Bowel Disease (IOIBD) began recommending that colitis sufferers avoid several of the additives discussed in this book. Dieticians and gastroenterologists are now urging patients to avoid additive-laden foods to ease bowel symptoms. It turns out that some of our digestive systems are trying to reject emulsifiers and other ubiquitous additives that are causing problems within our digestive tracts and well beyond. And yet most of the media—and the marketers who sell us "healthy" foods—haven't caught up. The United States Food and Drug Administration (FDA) has yet to act on a growing pile of evidence that those ingredients, even in "safe" amounts, can do us harm.

That mounting evidence is telling us what my patients were telling me for years, if only I had known how to hear them: some of the highly processed foods we eat are making us sick, and the restrictive diets that doctors tell their patients to try are difficult and only minimally helpful for far too many.

As I was writing this book, I considered how my patients asked me to tell them what they could eat instead of what they couldn't. I soon realized that they (and I) could eat everything—as long as most of it was real food, unadulterated by gut-roiling additives. If you seem to be struggling with your bowels, your blood sugar, your weight, or just not feeling right after you eat, and nothing seems to be helping very much, this book is for you. Even if you are just trying to eat healthfully but are tired of conflicting dietary advice that seems to change from year to year, this book is for you, too.

In part one, I will explain why certain food additives have become ubiquitous in what we eat, what they are doing to our microbiomes, and how this may be leading to astronomical levels of diet-related diseases. Part two was inspired by my patients asking me to tell them what to eat and is a practical guide to navigating the foods you may encounter throughout the day. In part three, I discuss how to navigate eating out, how to attempt to lose weight if that's a goal of yours, and how to troubleshoot specific issues that you might be facing. The end of the book includes some recipe ideas and a list of which additives to avoid so you can quickly review why they are best left on the shelf. We are all different, but we have something in common: we do much better when we eat real food.

Part I

Real Food Is Not the Enemy

Chapter 1

The Microbiome and the Rise of Diet-Related Diseases

Health is not valued till sickness comes.

—Thomas Fuller

Rodrigo is a fifty-two-year-old father of two grown children. He has been married for thirty years and has worked six days a week since he was a teenager. He attends church on his only day off each Sunday and manages to make it there some weekdays after work, too. He has worked in the construction industry in the US for more than twenty years, ever since immigrating from his native Honduras. His large biceps and thick forearms suggest that he still does a great deal of manual labor most of the day.

I ask anyway, "What do you do at work?"

Rodrigo smiles. "Whatever I have to," he replies and then expands on the answer.

He hauls lumber, pounds flooring, lays tile, paints. On weekends he spends a few more hours helping his parish priest with minor repairs to the church. Despite burning what must add up to hundreds of additional calories a day, his energy expenditure at his job equaling or exceeding the workouts of dedicated athletes, Rodrigo's gut hangs heavily over his belt. He has tested as having blood sugar in the diabetic range. He notes that a brother has type 2 diabetes, but no one in the older generation of his family does.

"No one?" I ask, just to be sure.

Rodrigo shakes his head. I go on to ask him what he eats. With the exception of dinner, which his wife prepares, he generally has gas station food for breakfast on the way to a job and prepreared sandwiches from the grocery store for lunch. He drinks energy drinks and sports drinks to help him keep going during the day. I ask what a typical dinner might be.

"We eat a lot of rice and beans," Rodrigo says, hanging his head. "I'm not supposed to, right?"

A coworker who had been diagnosed with diabetes a few years ago had told him to lay off the staples he was used to eating. Rodrigo told me that he had cut back a little on his portions, and he had switched to diet drinks as his friend had also advised. He had found that the convenience foods, however, were much harder to give up. While going through a review of various potential symptoms, Rodrigo admitted that he also had been having some bloating and gas.

"For how long?" I asked.

"Since I came to the US. I know it's from American food. People are always complaining about their stomach here."

But Rodrigo's intestinal upset wasn't going to kill him the way the diabetes might if left uncontrolled. Diabetes is a nefarious killer, chipping away at its victim's organs slowly; killing them quietly until the end when limbs are lost and days each week are spent on dialysis. But it is hard to consider that today's choices may lead to dialysis or death twenty years hence. The future is far away. For stressed, already overburdened people, it can be difficult to make choices today that may have no impact for years to come. Moreover, when people upend their lives to make changes and then don't see the results they were expecting, it can make them feel like it wasn't worth the effort. I could already sense Rodrigo's frustration building. He had been trying to follow what he thought were the rules, and yet here he was being told that he had diabetes anyway.

And, of course, Rodrigo wasn't alone. Across the country, rates of diabetes have been increasing year after year. Other conditions like metabolic syndrome and nonalcoholic fatty liver disease have only been identified within the past fifty years but already affect great swaths of the US population. Along with IBS, small intestinal bacterial overgrowth, and colon cancer, I'll refer to these as diet-related diseases, which are on the rise.

We need to start to dig a little deeper for answers as to why diet-related diseases are increasing so rapidly, and we'll start to do that in this chapter. But first, we have to stop blaming ourselves for these ailments. Your diagnosis isn't your fault.

It is easy, of course, to blame ill health on poor choices. Even when seemingly better explanations exist, we look askance at people who suffer with type 2 diabetes or high cholesterol or those who struggle with their weight. We conclude that they must be doing something wrong. Unfortunately, there is a long-standing precedent for doing so, and we don't need to go back terribly far in medical history to find a relevant example.

As recently as the 1990s, the medical establishment insisted that the cause of stomach ulcers was stress. When the Australian physician Barry Marshall correctly identified a bacterium, *Helicobacter pylori*, as the usual cause, no one would listen to him.[1] He became so frustrated by his colleagues that he proceeded to purposefully ingest a large quantity of the bacteria and cause ulcers in himself to prove his point. *H. pylori* is now recognized as the proximate cause of many ulcers and is treated with a two-week regimen of antibiotics. In 2005, Dr. Marshall, along with his pathologist coresearcher, received the Nobel Prize in Physiology or Medicine.

Dr. Marshall has further proposed that the cause of a lot of diseases that we can't figure out these days is likely to be bacterial or viral. It turns out that our bodies aren't temples; they are gardens, and our gardens can grow lovely, beneficial microorganisms (which we might refer to as good microorganisms) or treacherous weeds (bad microorganisms).

Our Microbiomes, Ourselves

Our microbiomes are suppsed to be our buddies. These gut bacteria (and some fungi and viruses) help with things that make intuitive sense, like our digestion, and things that until just recently hadn't even been considered, like our moods. But we don't fully understand them. So far, science has gotten around to thoroughly studying only a handful of the hundreds of organisms that make up our microbiomes (like bifidobacteria, which are among the most abundant; and lactobacilli, which were some of the first identified). The Human Microbiome Project is currently underway to try to understand what is going on in our guts,[2] but it turns out that mapping the microbiome is several magnitudes harder than mapping the human genome, where there is far less variation.

Human beings are remarkably biologically similar. Our microbiomes, not so much. There is a fair chance that while you share 99.9 percent of your DNA with your neighbor, you two might share only 10 percent of your microbial genomes.[3] In fact, your microbiome is profoundly different, not only from your neighbor's but also from what *your own microbiome looked like yesterday*, depending on what you ate. Just like different plants in a garden require specific fertilizers depending on the species you are trying to grow, bacteria and fungi in our microbiome grow or don't grow depending on what we feed them. And sometimes, they can start to work against us.

The bacteria in our guts are doing pretty much what we like to do. They're eating, hanging out, procreating, and producing by-products of digestion. Some of the bacteria are great members of our intestinal gardens and actually contribute to making our mucous lining better and stronger. Others outcompete the good guys for "land," and when there are too many of them or they don't get fed enough of the food they enjoy, they start consuming the lovely mucous. It turns out that a variety of diseases can be correlated to a dysbiosis (imbalance of microorganisms) in our guts.

The mucous is meant to keep bacteria, along with the fungi and viruses, in our guts where they belong. When it gets degraded by bacteria, elements of the microbiome may get too close to the actual cells making up our gastrointestinal (GI) tracts and may even get through them, triggering a reaction from the immune systems of genetically susceptible individuals.[4]

The by-products of bacterial digestion have been identified, and research is showing that there may be differences in what is being produced in the intestines of IBS sufferers compared with non-IBS sufferers.[5] There is also a difference in the microbiomes of people with obesity versus thin people and in people who have diabetes versus people who do not.[6]

Diet-Related Diseases and the Microbiome

If you are old enough to be reading this book, your body established its garden years ago. Perhaps unbeknownst to you, you've been planting and tending it since the day you were born. It is the product of your travels, your relationships, and even your hygiene habits. But it is mostly the result of what you've fed it. None of us is starting with virgin soil, and the combination of species growing is unique to each of us. And yet similarities emerge when we look at different diseases. To truly understand the interaction of what we eat (our fertilizers) and what we are growing (our microbiomes), let's look at what's going on in some of the most common diet-related diseases, starting with type 2 diabetes.

Type 2 Diabetes

Rodrigo had type 2 diabetes. While there are clearly genetic and possibly auto-immune components associated with type 2 diabetes, it is thought to be primarily a diet-related disease. That makes it unlike type 1 diabetes, which causes the body to stop producing insulin due to an autoimmune attack on the pancreas. According to the American Diabetes Association, nearly thirty-five million Americans, or 10.5 percent of the US population, has type 2 diabetes, while another eighty-eight million have prediabetes,[7] meaning they have trouble with their blood sugar and are at risk of developing diabetes in the next few years. For a point of comparison, in the 1950s, fewer than 1 percent of the US population had been diagnosed with diabetes.[8] While some of that might be attributable to less screening for diabetes and less accurate testing, a 1,000 percent increase in the past sixty years, with rates only expected to increase, should give us pause.

In type 2 diabetes, the body cannot make enough insulin to handle the amount of sugar in the blood, generally owing to a resistance to the hormone insulin. Insulin is involved in many chemical pathways in our bodies, but for the sake of simplicity, let's focus on its job of getting sugar (for fuel or storage) into our cells instead of floating around in our bloodstreams. When type 2 diabetes is developing, the tissues in the body become less sensitive to insulin, requiring more and more insulin for the needed blood sugar–lowering effect (a condition referred to as insulin resistance). In type 2 diabetes, the pancreas just can't keep up. It is not completely understood why some people develop insulin resistance—fat deposition in the abdomen is linked, though this may be a co-traveler and not the cause—but the connection to diet is undeniable.

Around the world, humans are consuming more and more sugar,[9] and increased sugar consumption has been named the culprit in the uptick in type 2 diabetes.[10] It is well known that reducing the amount of sugar and other carbohydrates one eats can help control diabetes. That was the only "treatment" available for generations before the advent of insulin injections and other medications.

But sugar isn't the only antagonist in the story of type 2 diabetes. Curiously, one study showed that diet sodas, which have no sugar and no calories, seem to increase the risk of developing diabetes just as much as the sugar-sweetened stuff.[11] Among scientists trying to puzzle this out, some are looking at the microbiome and changes that sweeteners like sucralose, stevia, and the polyols can induce in it.[12] Dietary emulsifiers and emulsifier-like additives (which we look at in detail in the next chapter) have also been implicated in changing the microbiome and perhaps promoting diabetes.[13] It turns out that whether some people develop problems with blood sugar may have something to do with what their microbiomes look like.

Certain bacterial species have been found to be more predominant in people with diabetes, while other bacteria have been shown to have some protective effect in perhaps preventing the development of the disease.[14] How carbohydrates are broken down, with subsequent effects on insulin resistance, has also been proposed as a contributor to the development of diabetes when certain bacterial species flourish.[15] Until we can sort out what an ideal microbiome should look like to prevent diabetes, we are left with diet, exercise, and medication as our available solutions.

The Metabolic Syndrome

When I was in medical school in the late 1990s learning about a poorly understood prediabetic condition in people who tended to gather weight around their waist, the condition was usually referred to as Syndrome X—a term coined in the late 1980s. The reason the condition was initially given such a mysterious name is that no one quite understood it. It seemed to lead to a higher risk of heart disease, and it was spreading through the population like wildfire. But it hadn't been recognized much before the late twentieth century. Besides weight gain around the middle of the body, people with Syndrome X tended to have high blood pressure, high blood sugar (though not quite to a level defined as diabetes), and a particular cholesterol profile where the good high-density cholesterol that protects against heart disease was very low and the triglycerides, which are the circulating fat in the blood, were very high.[16]

By the early 2000s, as the cluster of metabolic abnormalities became better understood and tens of millions of Americans were being diagnosed with it, the term *Syndrome X* fell out of favor. The condition would now be known by its more pedestrian and descriptive name—the metabolic syndrome—which today affects more than one-third of Americans.[17] The etiology of the syndrome, as discussed in the previous section, is thought to be abdominal weight gain leading to insulin resistance, as in type 2 diabetes. Since 2007, however, a new theory has emerged—one that originates in our intestines. Again, a disordered microbiome seems to be involved, leading to low-grade inflammation, which then leads to insulin resistance and its attendant metabolic consequences.[18]

Researchers conducted a study with mice where two widely used emulsifiers (additives) made up 1 percent of the study group's diet. These mice went on to develop a mouse version of the metabolic syndrome: they gained more weight, and had higher markers of inflammation and distinctive changes in their microbiomes compared to the control mice.[19] In other words, they looked a lot like us.

Other additives have been studied on human microbiome samples in the lab, and similar effects have been found.[20] In 2022, the researchers who investigated the emulsifiers' effects on mice published a study showing destructive changes to human participants' microbiomes when they consumed just one of the emulsifiers for only eleven days (more on this study in the next chapter).[21]

Nonalcoholic Fatty Liver Disease

A big change in our bodies has been in the rising development of nonalcoholic fatty liver disease (NAFLD), which can progress to nonalcoholic steatohepatitis (NASH) and then, in unfortunate cases, liver cirrhosis. Not only does cirrhosis from NASH cause liver failure, but 14 percent of people who develop cirrhosis from NASH will also develop liver cancer[22]—a potentially fatal diagnosis.

One-quarter of the US population is now thought to have NAFLD,[23] another diagnosis that did not exist until the 1980s.[24] It's indisputably a modern disease. Unlike diabetes or the metabolic syndrome, changes to the liver were diagnosed decades ago without blood work. Enlarged, yellowish livers, sometimes showing signs of scarring, were seen during surgery or on autopsies. However, in the past, those changes were usually associated with excess alcohol consumption. Now those changes are seen in people who don't drink (hence the name nonalcoholic fatty liver disease), and NAFLD is on track to become the leading cause of cirrhosis and liver failure in industrialized countries.[25]

The epidemic of NAFLD/NASH is most likely being driven by our modern, ultra-processed diets, but how?

NAFLD is usually seen in conjunction with the metabolic syndrome and diabetes. It has long been thought to be caused by insulin resistance and driven by excess caloric intake. Basically, when we have extra circulating fat in our bodies (not necessarily caused by eating fats, but often by eating carbohydrates), it goes into our liver to be stored for later use. The question now is why are some of those fat-storing livers becoming inflamed to the point that they are developing scarring and cirrhosis? After all, only a fraction of patients with NAFLD go on to develop the inflammation known as NASH and subsequent liver failure or perhaps liver cancer. Moreover, why is it that 10 to 15 percent of patients with fatty liver disease are considered to be of normal weight?[26]

This is where the microbiome may come into the picture again. Some bacteria can make a substance called lipopolysaccharide (LPS), which is a major component of their cell walls. It is also a potent stimulator of an inflammatory response by the immune system. LPS has been postulated as the trigger of the inflammation seen in a host of diseases, and researchers are discovering that the microbiomes of inflammatory disease sufferers seem to have more LPS-producing bacteria with resultant higher levels of LPS in the blood and higher markers of inflammation.[27] It turns out that the patients who progress to the inflammatory and cirrhotic phase of fatty liver disease have more of these LPS-producing bacteria, too.[28]

If we consider that dietary emulsifiers can break down the gut lining and allow for more contact with our gut bacteria or what they produce in other parts of our bodies (more on this later), it isn't hard to trace a path from a fatty to an inflamed liver.[29] That path may be even shorter for diseases mostly in our intestines.

Inflammatory Bowel Disease

The inflammatory bowel diseases (IBD) are mainly divided into ulcerative colitis (UC), which affects the large intestine and rectum; and Crohn's disease, which can affect the entire gastrointestinal tract. IBD is a devastating disease that can cause debilitating diarrhea, bleeding, and in the case of Crohn's disease, other complications in multiple organ systems. Many patients wind up having surgery to remove pieces of their GI tract. And IBD, too, may be getting more common because of our modern diets.

In 2015, three million people in the US had been diagnosed with either UC or Crohn's disease, a jump of one million people since 1999.[30] Another type of colitis called microscopic colitis affects fewer people, but its rates are also increasing. Like NAFLD, microscopic colitis didn't exist in the medical literature until the latter half of the twentieth century.[31] It's a modern phenomenon. Have we just developed better testing that makes diagnosing these diseases easier? The answer is yes, we have. There are blood tests that can suggest a diagnosis of IBD that didn't exist until fairly recently. But to get a definitive diagnosis, a biopsy of the intestines is still required. Perhaps we are performing biopsies on more people and picking up more cases, but a million more over fewer than twenty years? That's an awful lot to attribute to more aggressive testing.

Researchers in the US, France, and Germany have proposed that emulsifiers may be contributing to the increased incidences of colitis[32]—where the inflammation can get so severe that it becomes life-threatening. The mechanism behind this points directly to the disruption of the bacteria lining the intestinal wall and the subsequent degradation of the wall's protective mucous layer, leading to translocation (leakage) of gut bacteria outside of the intestines, provoking an inflammatory response by the body.[33] We'll return to this in the next chapter, but for now the key thing to keep in mind is that the microbiome is playing a large role once again.

Irritable Bowel Syndrome and Small Intestinal Bacterial Overgrowth

When I was a medical student, I attended a lecture given by a gray-haired professor of gastroenterology who declared that you weren't supposed to be aware of the organs contained within your abdomen. In his opinion, you should be able to go through your day unaware of what your stomach and intestines were doing. Like the circulation of your blood within veins and arteries or the movement of air through your lungs, the passage of food through your gastrointestinal system should be something that just happens mostly silently—so patients who had symptoms of bloating or pain should be evaluated for problems.

And yet throughout the years I've been a general internist, more and more people have arrived in my office telling me that not only are their bowels not being quiet; they are being downright disruptive. I've tested patients for myriad illnesses, including cancer and lactose intolerance, and have sent them to gastroenterologists and sometimes other specialists only to find that in many cases they were told there was nothing wrong. But how could that be right? My old professor had told me otherwise. These patients were highly aware of their bowels, so according to what I had been taught, something had to be abnormal.

By default these patients fell into the medical wastebasket diagnosis known as IBS. IBS is sometimes referred to as a functional disorder because we don't know exactly what causes it. We think something is wrong with the *functioning* of the GI system but can't quite find the piece of the immune system or infectious organisms that are responsible. While IBS isn't life-threatening in the way that IBD is, it can be life-altering for people who have it—they can have severe constipation or diarrhea or both.

Though the definition of IBS has changed slightly over the years, doctors follow standard guidelines to diagnose IBS. According to these guidelines, people need to have experienced the following symptoms for more than six months in total to be diagnosed with IBS: one day per week over the past three months of abdominal pain related to bowel movements, and a change in the frequency or form (or both) of their stool.[34]

Unfortunately, a lot of us fit these criteria. According to some experts, 15 to 20 percent of Americans are thought to be suffering with IBS, one of the highest rates in the world. This is compared with just a few percent of sufferers in Italy or France.[35]

Most IBS sufferers are classified as having IBS-M, or mixed IBS—they bounce between diarrhea and constipation. A significant percentage have IBS-D, with the *D* standing for diarrhea-predominant. Another group of sufferers have IBS-C, with, you guessed it, the *C* standing for constipation-predominant. But it is common for an IBS-D sufferer to have bouts of constipation and for an IBS-C sufferer to have occasional diarrhea.[36] IBS is one of the few diseases where one may have either or both. If its definition seems confusing, it's because it is. IBS is a poorly understood disorder, but it has become increasingly recognized as having its roots in a disordered gut.

While too many of the wrong types of gut bacteria may be the trigger for IBS and other diseases, sometimes what may be considered beneficial bacteria begin to proliferate in places they aren't supposed to. That condition often gets its own diagnosis—small intestinal bacterial overgrowth, or SIBO.

SIBO is a growing problem. Although it was barely mentioned when I was in medical school in the late 1990s, and then most often as a complication of some kind of intestinal malformation, upward of 15 percent of Americans may be suffering with this condition today.[37] Basically, SIBO is an excess of bacteria in the small intestine. No one is quite sure why this happens, but some blame medications that are used to control acid, dysfunctional immune systems, or even as a complication of popular weight-loss surgeries. While these possibilities certainly explain some cases, many people who do not use acid-blockers, seemingly have normal immune systems, and have never had gastrointestinal surgery are being diagnosed with SIBO. That these bacteria proliferate where they aren't meant to be in otherwise healthy people is another modern phenomenon.

Bacterial overgrowth is one suspected cause of IBS symptoms.[38] SIBO presents with many symptoms that overlap with IBS, such as bloating, abdominal discomfort, and diarrhea. It has been well documented that bacteria in IBS patients can migrate from the large intestine and set up shop in the small intestine, where they are not supposed to be.[39] There are several hypotheses that have been formulated around why this may happen in some individuals and not others, but it is clear that too many bacteria in the wrong place can cause problems. Overlap with IBS is thought to be as high as 78 percent in one well-done study, and half of the patients with IBS experienced resolution of their symptoms after being treated for SIBO.[40]

SIBO is typically treated with a short course of antibiotics and longer courses of different antibiotics when it commonly returns. Increasingly, it has been suggested that IBS be treated with similar antibiotics.[41] But dosing with antibiotics is carpet-bombing our intestines—taking out the good bacteria along with the bad. Indeed, some patients who have IBS believe their symptoms started after a course of antibiotics. Manipulating our microbiomes with antibiotics can have dramatic effects on which bacteria proliferate, and that has a great effect on how some guts wind up behaving. With antibiotic treatment, we are generally just hoping to get rid of more of the bad guys than the good guys. It's like using a powerful weed killer in our gardens and hoping it doesn't damage the plants we'd like to flourish.

Colon Cancer

It is becoming established science that the microbiomes of people who develop colon cancer are different from those who do not. It turns out that some bacteria produce more of what the colon cancer cells use to facilitate their growth. Other bacteria may produce substances that impede growth.[42] Scientists are just beginning to sort out which bacteria may be involved in the development of colon cancer.

What is clear is that while colon cancer used to be thought of as an older person's disease, it no longer is. In 2019, the Boston-based Dana-Farber Cancer Institute established the Young-Onset Colorectal Cancer Center specifically for patients under age fifty, who they note have increased by 51 percent

Sorting the Good Guys from the Bad

The idea that bacteria can be beneficial is pretty new. It represents a pendulum swing in the opposite direction of several decades of medical practice and public health, where it was thought that eliminating bacteria would make us all healthier. Under this old and debunked paradigm, bacteria were bad, and getting rid of them was an unabashed good. Antibiotics have saved countless lives by vanquishing pathogenic bacteria from our bodies. But taking an antibiotic at the first sign of sinus pressure, blasting all of the bacteria in our bodies, leads to other problems.

We now recognize that many types of bacteria work in a commensal relationship with our bodies and are indeed good. The problem is that we have a shaky understanding of which bacteria these may be and a worse understanding of *where* they should be. We have a fairly good understanding of many of the bacteria that can cause harm, and rightfully treat them when they make us ill, but less of an understanding of those that are good for us.

Complicating matters further is that the more than one-hundred-year-old system for organizing bacteria into broad categories is mostly based on how the bacteria look, not on what they do. For example, *Escherichia coli*, *E. coli* for short, make up a great deal of our healthy fecal matter. But one type of *E. coli*, O157:H7, is responsible for many cases of foodborne illness and even death. *E. coli* species also seem to be elevated in types of inflammatory bowel disease—otherwise known as colitis.[43] And yet, other studies report that types of *E. coli* are protective against bad bacteria and perhaps helpful in inflammatory bowel disease.[44]

All *E. coli* are certainly not created equal. But this is the classification system we have. When you hear that Bacteroidetes are good bacteria or Firmicutes are bad bacteria, remember that this is an overly simplistic way of categorizing the organisms. We are still sorting out the good from the bad.[45] (This will be particularly important when we talk about probiotic supplements—more on that in a later chapter.)

since 1994. The rates of colon and rectal cancer among young people are now increasing so rapidly that by 2030, they are expected to double and quadruple respectively.[46]

Baffling the doctors and researchers is the fact that the young victims of colon cancer have no easily identifiable risk factors—they don't smoke more, they don't experience obesity at higher rates, and they usually don't have other conditions that would predispose someone to cancer. So scientists are increasingly looking toward diet as a potential culprit. They are finding that eating highly processed food in general confers an increased risk of cancer.[47] Consuming certain emulsifiers, specifically, may increase the risk of colon cancer.[48]

Failed Solutions: Making Real Food the Enemy

Since our bodies are gardens (not temples), let's begin by examining our gardens from the ground up: genetic predisposition (our soil) is combined with not-so-friendly bacteria (the invasive weeds) and certain food additives (fertilizer that encourages the weeds), and are wreaking havoc on our bodies. The idea that food plays a major role in our health isn't new. Rodrigo had been getting the message for twenty years that what he had been eating wasn't agreeing with him.

It might be a good place here to pause and say that I made sure that Rodrigo didn't have colon cancer or another condition, and if you are suffering with any symptoms, you should get a full workup from a physician. Get a diagnosis and make sure nothing else is going on before you turn to any book for advice—dietary or otherwise.

Even though Rodrigo had already suspected that his diet was not ideal, the first place he thought he should make changes, besides cutting back on regular sodas, was in the traditional rice and beans he was eating. His friend with diabetes had been counseled to do just that.

It makes sense that some proposed solutions to diet-related diseases focus on changing what we eat. However, for the past several decades, we've clung to the traditional teaching that if you have stomach trouble or diabetes or are gaining weight, the problem lies with carbohydrates or fats or perhaps the calories you are consuming. That means we're still relying on certain restrictive diets—many of which are, unfortunately, only minimally effective but are still being recommended by health professionals. Let's take a closer look at a few.

Low-FODMAP Diet

Digestion of food occurs throughout the gastrointestinal tract, starting with the mouth, proceeding to the stomach, the small intestine, and then through to the large intestine. At each step food is broken down further and further into usable components. Traditional teaching tells us that various enzymes contained throughout the gastrointestinal tract break down different substances that we eat, and the stuff that can't be broken down winds up in our colon and then bulks up our poop. From that understanding, which isn't wrong, just incomplete, researchers at Monash University in Australia came up with the low-FODMAP diet, which is often recommended not only to patients with IBS, but also to others suffering from a variety of ailments.[49]

As I mentioned in the introduction, FODMAP is shorthand for fermentable oligosaccharides, disaccharides, monosaccharides, and polyols. *Oligosaccharides*, *disaccharides*, and *monosaccharides* are fancy terms describing sugars (saccharides) by the number of basic sugar structures they contain (oligo- [few], di- [two], and mono- [one]) that we can have trouble digesting. The polyols are sugar alcohols that find their way into a host of food products as low-calorie sweeteners and coatings that may prove difficult to digest, especially when in combination with other carbohydrates.[50]

The science explaining the difficulty of digesting some FODMAPs is reliable, as is the bloating, discomfort, and abnormal bowel movements people can have when eating hard-to-digest foods, so avoiding them makes sense. FODMAPs abound in processed foods. However, whole foods, like chickpeas and sweet potatoes, that contain FODMAPs also contain important longer chain sugar-like substances that we know as complex carbohydrates and starches. And adherents of the low-FODMAP diet are told to avoid even the healthy whole foods (at least in the beginning), which might be a needlessly restrictive and complicated approach for many.

The low-FODMAP diet was originally proposed by researchers asking which foods caused people to have gastrointestinal upset. Lactose, or dairy intolerance, had long been noted. So, too, had flatulence caused by legumes. Recall the old ditty *beans, beans, good for your heart. The more you eat, the more you fart.* While surely not the most beautiful poetry, something must be said for its accuracy.

A large nutrition study found that people who consumed a diet rich in legumes (beans) had less heart disease, so that part is certainly true.[51] As for the second sentence, well, I probably don't have to tell you that eating beans might make you gassy. The excess gas produced by the fiber-digesting bacteria in our microbiome has been proposed as being partly responsible for the bloating that most IBS patients have. Thus, the diet says to get rid of the fermentable oligosaccharides, which are in beans, wheat, garlic, onions, and broccoli, along with a host of other fruits and vegetables.

Among other things, the low-FODMAP diet has been criticized for restricting fiber intake.[52] Fiber is supposed to be good for us. Eating enough of it is supposed to be the key to success in the bathroom. It helps lower cholesterol and is thus thought to lower the risk of heart disease (*beans, beans, good for your heart...*). It is supposed to make us feel full and maybe even help control blood sugar.[53] But we don't actually digest the fiber—our gut bacteria do. When our microbiomes digest fiber and other substances, besides producing gas they make short-chain fatty acids, which can affect myriad bodily processes in a positive way (see the box). So we don't want to starve our microbiomes, but we don't want to feed them the wrong things, either.

The first thing to recognize is that fiber is not necessarily good in isolation. A fiber is a substance, usually a long-chain carbohydrate molecule, that the body cannot digest. It's food for our microbiome, and there are lots of different kinds. When fiber-like additives are added to ultra-processed foods as emulsifiers and thickeners, the additives may be feeding the wrong bacteria or possibly bacteria in the wrong places (I'm looking at you, SIBO). How healthy what we are eating is for us may depend in large part on what our microbiome does with what is provided to it and where in the gut this happens.

A great deal of our gut microbiome resides in our colon, the part of the intestines that extends from the small intestine to the end and is responsible for a lot more than we used to suppose. But our microbiome exists throughout our GI tract, and additives that we can't break down are served up to them as sustenance. Unfortunately, these additives don't often make it on to the FODMAP diet's what-to-avoid lists, which focuses, I believe misguidedly for many of us, on whole, real foods. Researchers who have pooled the results of several studies done on IBS patients following low-FODMAP diets found only a modest reduction in symptoms such as bloating, abdominal pain, and diarrhea.[54]

"Anti-Inflammatory" Diets

The evidence is mounting for a connection between noncommunicable diseases (meaning diseases we don't transmit from person to person) and the functioning of the microbiome, with recent findings of disruptive microbiomes in rheumatoid arthritis,[55] depression,[56] and even heart disease.[57] Heightened or disordered inflammation is often a commonly cited link between the various ailments.

People will ask me if eating a so-called anti-inflammatory diet might help their specific condition. It has been shown that when people consume large quantities of sugar, the inflammatory markers in their blood increase.[58] Red meat consumption has also been implicated in inflammatory disease.[59] In general, however, it is challenging to show that a particular food increases (or decreases) inflammation in the body. But studies are showing that dietary patterns, like consuming large quantities of ultra-processed foods, can lead to inflammation and inflammatory diseases.[60] Some popular health gurus, however, have encouraged

Short-Chain Fatty Acids

When different bacterial species digest what we feed them, they make molecules called short-chain fatty acids (SCFAs). There are several different kinds of SCFAs made by bacteria as they consume fermentable foods from our diet, depending on what we are eating and which bacteria are doing the digesting in our guts. How much, or even if, bacteria produce certain SCFAs is also dependent on what else is in the intestinal environment, including carbohydrates, gases, and minerals.[61]

Different SCFAs have varying effects on our bodies. The cells in our colons can use some of the SCFAs as energy themselves. SCFAs are also used as signaling molecules to tell a variety of cells in our bodies what to do (although one might argue that the bacteria are actually telling us what to do since they are making the SCFAs ... but I wouldn't suggest dwelling on that for too long). Two of the SCFAs can stimulate hormones that tell us we are full. Liver cells, nerve cells, muscle cells, and immune cells also have receptors to receive signals from SCFAs.[62] Some SCFAs have even been shown to inhibit cancer cells.[63]

people to avoid specific whole foods based on more dubious claims, such as the notion that nightshades (like tomatoes, peppers, and eggplant) or foods that contain lectins (proteins found in legumes) are bad for the gut. Meanwhile, the data actually support eating patterns, like the Mediterranean and DASH (a diet designed to reduce blood pressure) diets, which embrace whole foods and emphasize a wide variety of fruits and vegetables, as being truly anti-inflammatory and disease-preventing.[64]

If you've found that avoiding tomatoes or beans seems to help you, by all means, don't eat them. But the question we need to ask is why these natural foods are a problem when we've gone generations without whole foods causing these issues. Consider the advice Rodrigo heard to limit his intake of rice and beans. While limiting the amount of white rice he was consuming wasn't terrible advice, Rodrigo's grandmother was eating that just fine (as are grandparents around the world). The older people in Honduras did not seem to suffer from the same maladies his generation and his children's generation were dealing with. They worked hard, but so did he. Yet they ate very differently. While his friends in Honduras were just as likely as he was to tear open a package of something for lunch, his grandmother was still butchering her own chickens. She didn't consider Rodrigo's typical meals as food at all. And according to Rodrigo, she didn't have any serious health problems.

It is important to consider that many of the diseases we've discussed in this chapter barely existed before the advent of many of the additives we are consuming today. Some foods do seem to be more inflammatory than others, but perhaps if our intestinal linings weren't being torn up by emulsifiers and similar additives, the foods would remain quiescent in our intestines as they have for hundreds of years.

Finding the Real Culprits

The fact is, humans have been consuming beans and broccoli for a long time, but the rates of IBS, diabetes, and other diet-related diseases have been increasing just in the past few decades. While there hasn't been an explosion in fruit and vegetable intake in the US in the last several decades, there has been a big increase in the ingestion of ultra-processed foods.[65] What if the low-FODMAP diet has the right idea—that some food items are just really difficult for certain humans to digest—but the wrong list for many of us? What if we've been mistakenly blaming real foods for what the food *additives* are doing?

As a physician, I will be the first to point out that correlation does not equal causation—meaning that it is hard to prove a direct cause-and-effect relationship when we study populations. It took scientists decades to directly link lung cancer to smoking, though that connection seems obvious today. So although additive consumption has increased in the past several decades, one might point out that use of computers, our sedentary lifestyle, and perhaps levels of stress have also increased. Why couldn't any of these or hundreds of other lifestyle factors be the cause of the explosion in our modern maladies?

Well, they could be, and we should study them. Ideally, we should study everything that could be contributing to our ill health. But that's going to take a lot of time and a lot of money. In the meantime, there are millions of Americans and millions more around the globe struggling with health issues that were much rarer a few decades ago and are much less prevalent in the parts of the world not consuming a Western diet. We are getting diseases, like colon cancer, at younger and younger ages that were formerly seen in the middle-aged and old.[66] Right now, a lot of the signals are pointing to our ultra-processed diets as the chief source of our declining health.

Our intestinal landscape, microorganisms, and the food they encounter all matter. We really are what we eat. And according to some scientists, what we are eating sometimes shouldn't even be considered food—at least not for us. In the next chapter, we'll look at promoters of intestinal weeds, namely, those additives that are disrupting our microbiomes.

Chapter 2

What's Gone Wrong with Our Food?

It's the little details that are vital. Little things make big things happen.

—John Wooden

Linda is a thirty-year-old personal trainer. She thinks she eats pretty healthfully—no fast food and very little in the way of sweets. And she is fastidious about her appearance and hygiene. Her long hair has been meticulously blown straight, and her understated makeup has been deftly applied, making her beauty appear effortless. She confides in hushed tones that she is in my office for what she believes is a rash on her behind, which in the past few weeks has been getting worse. She thinks it might have something to do with getting sweaty when she exercises but notes that nothing much has changed in her routine.

I have Linda change, then I drape a sheet over her lower half and ask her to lie down on the examination table. Upon examining the aforementioned area, it is clear that she is having a reaction to something her skin is coming into contact with. The skin is so raw that it has begun to peel. I'm surprised that she waited as long as she did to come in.

When she's back in her clothes, I ask Linda what products she is using on that area—soaps, detergents, anything different at all? Linda's cheeks flush crimson. "When I poop, it's just so messy," she confides. She tells me that several times a day, she moves her bowels and finds that she can't get clean without using disposable wipes. She has even taken to carrying a pack in her purse.

I ask Linda to opt for wet toilet paper to clean herself instead, and she looks crestfallen.

"Isn't everyone's poop like that?" she asks.

Her voice is so quiet that I am not sure I heard her correctly. I confirm that she is asking me what a normal poop is. She is.

"There's a big range of normal," I tell her. But what she was describing didn't seem to be it.

We tested her stool and did some blood work. Linda also had a colonoscopy. All her results were within normal ranges. Linda's bowel problem didn't rise to the level of a serious disease, but it was enough to disrupt her life. Linda told me that she was trying to eat more fiber, which upon further questioning seemed to come in the form of fiber additives in packaged food bars. She had seen no improvement in her problem. And Linda wasn't the only patient telling me things like this. Over the past ten years, I've noticed that many more people have been trying to cope with really strange bowel movements.

I suspected that despite spending hours a week working toward good health, Linda was being undone by a diet she had been told would be healthy. Still, she was uncertain about changing her diet and taking a break from her additive-laden bars. Was I sure the food she was eating was the cause of her troubles? I couldn't promise her with 100 percent certainty (I always try to think of what else could be going on—the hallmark of being an internal medicine physician), but I thought it was worth a try based on what I'd been seeing in other patients and in myself.

In medicine, you need to satisfy a concept called biologic plausibility—meaning that even if something seems like it is the cause of a disease, you have to be able to explain why that is the case in an individual. What was the reason these seemingly innocuous substances could be causing problems in me and in some of my patients but hadn't shown up in the studies that approved them as food additives in the first place?

My experience during my years as an internal medicine physician helped me with that piece of the puzzle. Over the course of two decades in medicine, I have seen so-called miracle drugs unveiled and then pulled from the market. Their removal mostly followed a familiar pattern. In early studies, minor or few problems were noted. Then when the drug was released for use by the wider public,

32

unforeseen problems arose. There are many reasons for why this might happen, but it usually comes down to one or more of three possibilities.

First, drug research, like food additive research, is generally sponsored by the producer of the substance. Practically, this means that a lot of studies that paint the product in a bad light are never actually published.

Second, the studies are done in small groups of people over short periods of time. Sometimes an effect isn't seen until more people are looked at, or sometimes it takes a longer exposure to a substance to develop problems with it. Some studies are just too small or too short to pick up problems.

Third, drugs are rarely studied in combination with other drugs. The same goes for additives. So while a drug may have no or minimal untoward effects in isolation, when combined, we see what are called drug-drug interactions that produce effects that no one could have predicted. It is possible that by combining multiple food additives, which disrupt the intestines in different ways, we are winding up with health issues the one additive by itself would not have caused.

That third possibility is key here. A typical meal, even a so-called healthy one in the US, might easily contain a half-dozen fillers, emulsifiers, and softening agents. In isolation and eaten in small quantities, maybe one of these additives wouldn't cause trouble, but they aren't eaten in isolation or even in small amounts anymore. And our gastrointestinal system isn't being exposed to the substances for five or seven or even thirty days as they were in the studies that were done to approve them. Our bowels have been trying to digest these additives for decades now. What happens when you mix a little something that feeds the wrong kind of gut bacteria, with a little something that induces gut inflammation, with a little something that disrupts the intestinal lining? It is conceivable that you begin to create a gut environment that promotes problems.[67]

The Rise of Ultra-Processed "Food"

Carlos Monteiro, MD, PhD, a professor of nutrition and public health at the University of São Paulo in Brazil and a member of the World Health Organization Nutrition Guidance Expert Advisory Group, is credited with coining the term and defining just what an ultra-processed food is. He suggests that we look at most ultra-processed food additives as chemical compounds that are not food. According to Dr. Monteiro, "Ultra-processed foods are not modified foods. They really do not contain foods."[68]

Among health gurus and adherents of certain diets, it's become trendy to bash processed foods. But humans have been processing food for a long time. The first human who dried a piece of meat or salted the fish they had caught was also processing food—in other words, changing it from its original form, usually to preserve it. We've been canning, pickling, and fermenting foods to strengthen our food supply for thousands of years. Humans probably got where we are today, in part, by figuring out how to process food. (Eating food that's gone rotten or starving for lack of food are not particularly good ways to sustain a society.)

Just how we process food, however, has changed a lot in the last few decades. Consider the simple loaf of bread. Anyone who has baked bread knows it is a time-consuming task. There's usually a lot of kneading and waiting around for the bread to rise. A good sourdough bread needs a day or even longer to develop its flavor and texture. Commercial bread bakeries don't have that kind of time. So to quickly bake many loaves, a team of British chemists developed the Chorleywood method in the 1960s. It substitutes enzymes, emulsifiers, and "dough improvers" for the protein bonding and rising that naturally occur in bread processing—taking a processed food like bread and making it into an ultra-processed product that needs additional ingredients to make it taste and act like bread.[69]

As another example, take the now common ingredient xanthan gum, which was first discovered in the 1960s. This emulsifier helps thicken foods and prevents separation. By the 1990s, it had been joined by several other food gums.[70] Together with a host of other additives, the possibilities to get ever more creative with processed foods appeared endless. And so the 1960s marked the beginning of America's love of ultra-processed foods, with many other countries quickly adopting elements of the ultra-processed diet within the next generation.[71]

In terms of food processing technology, we've gone from a horse and buggy to a Ferrari in the past fifty years. Only our fancy-food sports car doesn't have any safety features built in. We are speeding down the culinary superhighway at 120 miles per hour without seat belts or a reliable steering system, and, quite frankly, our tires aren't attached all that well. The regulations for our new technology are based on the simple techniques we used to use (which wouldn't need a whole lot in the way of regulation), not the sleek products lining the supermarket aisles.

Just as we can't adequately use the language of the horse-drawn carriage to explain how a modern engine works, a new way of talking about our food supply was needed. Dr. Monteiro decided to tackle the problem of how we talk about our new food supply by developing what he calls the Nova classification system. *Nova*, which means "new" in Portuguese, is increasingly gaining in popularity to better describe how we eat today by dividing food into four categories.

Category one is primarily made up of whole foods and foods that are minimally processed, so both an apple and dried apples would make it into this category. White rice and brown rice would also both be category one foods.

Category two foods are culinary ingredients used to prepare other foods. Cooking oils and salt would fall into this category. You are unlikely to eat them on their own or use them in great quantities if doing your own food preparation. They are the sidekicks of category one foods.

Category three foods are what we think of as traditionally processed foods. Bread and cheese would be considered processed, having been changed from their original forms of wheat and milk (which would be in category one had they not been processed).

To the great dismay of children (and many adults) everywhere, you cannot have a diet consisting of just bread and cheese. They probably should be eaten in moderation, but the constituent ingredients in these foods, and other processed foods, can typically be easily recognized. That is, *if* they haven't been ultra-processed—meaning if they haven't had processes and additives added to them that save the manufacturer time and money but introduce substances to our food that our bodies may not be prepared to handle. And chances are if you are reading this in the US or increasingly in many other countries around the world, your bread and cheese might have a lot of those extra substances, which would push those previously merely processed foods into the fourth category in the Nova system.

The ultra-processed foods make up the fourth category proposed by Dr. Monteiro and was adopted into the Dietary Guidelines for the Brazilian Population in 2015. Scientists around the world have embraced this new language to help us talk about what we are actually eating today.[72] According to the guidelines, "Breads and baked goods become ultra-processed foods when, in addition to wheat flour, yeast, water, and salt, their ingredients include substances such as hydrogenated vegetable fat, sugar, starch, whey, emulsifiers, and other additives."[73]

Nova Food Classification System

Category 1	Whole foods or minimally processed foods	*Examples:* Brown or white rice, fresh apples or dried apples
Category 2	Culinary ingredients (items used in small amounts to prepare foods)	*Examples:* Cooking oils, salt, spices
Category 3	Traditionally processed foods	*Examples:* Traditionally made breads and cheeses, pasta
Category 4	Ultra-processed foods	*Examples:* Most commercially made breads, most packaged ice creams, crackers, margarine

Dr. Monteiro explained to me that for most of human history and also in the history of medicine, we were coping with diseases of deprivation—too little nutrition brought about many of our maladies—so that's what we focused on. Now we are mostly faced with different problems. A typical internal medicine doctor will see several patients with diet-related diseases each day. Only in many countries today, they aren't diseases of deprivation—at least not in the way we have thought about it in the past. Times have changed. How we think about disease has been slow to catch up.

"With the advent of ultra-processed foods, the range of mechanisms [for how we get chronic diseases] increased a lot," Dr. Monteiro says. "It isn't only to do with the nutrient imbalance in food, but also how these products are manufactured—highly technological products—requires additives that are only used by these big corporations. They are [making] re-engineered foods. When you use extrusion by high temperatures, you generate new substances. You create 'xeno-biotics,' which is any substance in a food that does not belong in food. They are strange and they are strange to our metabolism. Our diet starts to affect our health, not just because of the nutrients, but because of the other substances. This is what characterizes the fourth group of Nova."[74]

Could my patients' feeling better on whole-food diets be due to their lim-iting or eliminating ultra-processed, category-four foods? After talking with Dr. Monteiro, it seemed highly likely. And, I realized, I'd been seeing this in my patients with diabetes for years.

The endocrinologists and dieticians I had worked with in Boston had taught me to try to get patients with diabetes to limit their carbohydrate intake to no more than 150 grams per day, so I had been recommending this for many years. For patients who could do it, it absolutely helped. But a lot of my patients also needed insulin therapy to lower their blood sugar to a level that would help pro-tect their organs from the ravages of diabetes. Besides the cost, the inconvenience and fear of injections caused many of my patients to balk at getting injections. They insisted there must be something else they could do. So along with advising they limit carbohydrate intake, I also started advising them to get rid of highly processed foods.

For some, this was much easier than for others. For those who had come to the US more recently and had experienced more scratch cooking at home, I needed to do little more than tell them to eat natural food. These patients nod-ded and told me about soup recipes full of vegetables, bean dishes, and chicken that I imagined falling off the bone. They promised to stick to these meals.

I hoped for the best, but I had been taught that diet wouldn't do enough for patients whose blood sugar was out of control. I was convinced we would be starting insulin injections in a few months when my patients didn't see the change in their blood work they had hoped for.

I started doing this a few years ago, and what happened next still amazes me when I look at patient lab results today. A normal measure of blood sugar over time, called the hemoglobin A1C, should be less than 5.7 percent in some-one without blood sugar problems. We try to keep it less than 7 percent in most patients with diabetes. Many of the patients I first treated had hemoglobin A1C levels that were 12 or 13 percent, which would normally automatically trigger starting insulin injections. And, indeed, if my patients had been amenable to them (read: able to afford it), I would have prescribed injections immediately. Instead, they started taking older oral medications, and they began eating fewer carbohydrates, mostly eliminating those from ultra-processed sources. After three or four months, I had to squint when the blood work of those who began to focus on whole foods came back. Their hemoglobin A1C levels had dropped as if they had been on insulin—they were now at 6, 7, and sometimes 8 percent. Not all were at their goal yet, but I had been taught a response this dramatic without insulin injections was impossible. Certainly not everyone was able to avoid using insulin, but I had been taught that if the hemoglobin A1C was in the double digits, insulin therapy was unavoidable (at least without some of the newer medications that arrived on the market a few years ago and were unaffordable for my patients without insurance).

Most of these patients still needed at least one oral diabetes medication, so just eating whole foods isn't a cure. (I advise talking with your doctor before attempting to make any changes in your diet or medication regimen if you have diabetes.) But it is undeniable that getting rid of additive-laden foods makes a huge difference.

The Additive Invasion

By law, ingredients have to be listed on packaged food. Not so when we go out to eat, but at least when preparing food at home, we have more control over what goes into our bodies. The problem is that most consumers just don't know a lot about additives.

Though food additives have to be approved for use by the FDA, there is a fair amount of disagreement over what should be allowed and what shouldn't. Countries all over the world have their versions of FDA all looking at the same scientific evidence about the same additives we are using, and yet sometimes they reach very different conclusions.

How can this be if everyone is looking at the same data? Many times the root of the disagreements is that the science around food additives isn't particularly strong. This then leaves a great deal of room for values to enter into the interpretation of the data. In the US, particularly for additives that were approved many decades ago, unless the evidence is unequivocally bad, the attitude seems to be to leave well enough alone. In Europe, it is somewhat similar, though there might be a bit more skepticism on the part of European regulators.

We can see this difference exemplified by looking at how the FDA defines a food additive versus how the European Food Safety Authority (EFSA) does.

A food additive is defined in Section 201(s) of the FD&C [Federal Food, Drug, and Cosmetic] Act as any substance the intended use of which results or may reasonably be expected to result, directly or indirectly, in its becoming a component or otherwise affecting the characteristic of any food (including any substance intended for use in producing, manufacturing, packing, processing, preparing, treating, packaging, transporting, or holding food; and including any source of radiation intended for any such use); if such substance is not GRAS [generally recognized as safe] or sanctioned prior to 1958 or otherwise excluded from the definition of food additives.

The FDA makes room for a lot of exceptions by excluding GRAS substances from its definition of a *food additive*, which it says is "any substance that is intentionally added to food … that is subject to premarket review and approval by FDA, unless the substance is generally recognized, among qualified experts, as having been adequately shown to be safe under the conditions of its intended use, or unless the use of the substance is otherwise exempted from the definition of a food additive." In fact, the notation at the end of the FDA webpage makes sure to state that there are other exceptions not listed in this short definition.[75]

In contrast, the European agency simply has this to say about food additives: "[A food additive is] any substance not normally consumed as a food in itself and not normally used as a characteristic ingredient of food whether or not it has nutritive value, the intentional addition of which to food for a technological purpose results in it or its by-products becoming directly or indirectly a component of such foods."

The European agency then goes on to list many categories of food additives, some of which are as follows:[76]

- Anti-caking agent
- Anti-foaming agent
- Bulking agent
- Color
- **Emulsifier**
- Firming agent
- Flavor enhancer
- Flour treatment agent
- Foaming agent
- **Gelling agent**

- Glazing agent
- Humectant
- **Modified starch**
- Preservative
- Raising agent
- Sequestrant
- **Stabilizer**
- **Sweetener**
- **Thickener**

The ones in bold are the types of additives we will pay special attention to in this book, because the specific additives that have been shown to be microbiome-altering and inflammation-producing belong to these categories.

Whereas the European regulatory agencies attempt to be as inclusive as possible, the USFDA readily excludes substances as food additives and their subsequent regulation. European values are to err ever so slightly on the side of protecting individuals and perhaps harming industry even in the face of weak data. US regulatory values seem to come down more on the side of industry. (For more on the history of regulation of additives in the US, I recommend *The Poison Squad* by Deborah Blum.)

It wasn't always this way. Once upon a time and not so long ago, foods like breads and cheeses had to be clearly labeled if they had been adulterated with ingredients that wouldn't ordinarily be added to these foods. In 1938, with the rise of store-bought processed foods, the FDA declared that the packaging of food products should clearly state if it contains imitation ingredients. In 1973, after much lobbying effort from the food industry, the FDA reversed this rule. And after several decades, emulsifiers and additives were slipped into a great number of foods that never had them.[77] There would be no reason to limit the quantity of additives in our food if they were completely safe, after all.

All of this was done quietly. A popular drink that would have been labeled *Chocolate Flavored* became just *Chocolate*, even as the amount of non-cocoa ingredients increased. The front of a yogurt container that contains any number of fillers and emulsifiers looks pretty much identical to a container of yogurt that is made entirely of cultured milk. Today, without a detailed exploration of an ingredient list, most consumers have no idea what they are eating.

Soy Lecithin: An Unexpected Upside?

Soy lecithin may have one added benefit: It's a good way to baby-step your way into label reading. If you are planning to eat something that's labeled "Contains Soy" that otherwise shouldn't—like bread or cookies—it's a fair bet the food item contains soy lecithin along with a host of other additives. Because soy is an allergen that can induce a severe reaction in someone with a true soy allergy (not just with an intolerance to it), the ingredient is often bolded and more obvious on the packaging than other food additives. But beware. Lecithins are now being derived from sunflowers and other sources. It's not the soy that is the problem for people without a soy allergy; it's the lecithin. And no matter where the lecithin comes from, it is still basically the same chemical compound doing the same emulsifying job with the same potential side effects.

Untangling the Emulsifier Mystery

The reasoning that has been promoted for decades by scientists, marketers, and ultimately by the ultra-processed food industry is, if the food or substance that the additive comes from is safe, why shouldn't the additive be? The burden to prove safety is therefore not terribly high anywhere, and it is up to the scientific community to prove that it is *un*safe. The funding to do so is difficult to come by.

Many of the substances currently in wide use were approved years ago after small rodent studies and possibly testing on just handfuls of healthy young adults.

Researchers have determined that of all of the additives used in food products in the US, only about 21 percent of them "have feeding studies necessary to estimate a safe level of exposure"[78] to the additive. There seems to have been a plan at the FDA in the 1980s to rectify this, but that never came to fruition.[79] Today, these additives are being ingested by tens, if not hundreds, of millions of people on a daily basis. And they are being ingested with a host of other substances. Laying blame on any particular additive for one disease or another presents a great challenge to researchers. It is going to take a while—possibly a decade or more—for them to gather enough data to satisfy regulators.

Emulsifiers are a particular category of additives that have been used in food for decades. They are called surfactants when used in food or pharmaceuticals and detergents when used in cleaning products.[80] Their main purpose is to get oil and water to mix and stay mixed. While consumers may flock to items that claim to be preservative-free or as having no artificial colors, food purveyors are under no pressure to attempt to make their foods free of emulsifiers. They are distinctly different from other additives and most of us don't know what they are or what they are doing in our food. Thinking of an emulsifier as a detergent is helpful because we've all seen how those work—there's a part that is attracted to water and a part that is attracted to fat (or grease, if you will).

Thickening agents, stabilizers, and modified starches are separate categories (see the EFSA list on page 40), but they are often used in conjunction with emulsifiers and are essentially doing a lot of the same work. For the sake of simplicity, I often use the word *emulsifier* as a catch-all for the additives that blend and stabilize ultra-processed foods; a few common ones you may encounter on food packaging include carrageenan, mono- and diglycerides, and polysorbate. By combining emulsifiers with newly discovered thickening and stabilizing agents, processed food purveyors created myriad foods that could last longer on supermarket shelves while giving consumers the illusion of freshness and the added benefit of cheaper food. In one review from 2019, it was estimated that up to half of the food we eat contains one or more of these additives, and yet the authors challenged that "remarkably, there has been little study of the potential harmful effects of ingested detergents or emulsifiers in humans."[81] But there are researchers who are trying.

Benoit Chassaing, PhD, at France's National Institute of Health and Medical Research, *Institut National de la Santé et de la Recherche Médicale* (INSERM), is studying twenty individual emulsifiers one by one. Dr. Chassaing's lab exposed bacteria in typical human feces to each of the twenty emulsifiers to look for an effect on the bacteria's growth. Most of the emulsifiers (though not all) altered the microbiome in an unfavorable way.[82] Since the project was begun with healthy donors, Dr. Chassaing is now planning to expand this study to look at what happens to the microbiomes of people with various diet-related ailments.

"It is very important to understand the variation in humans," Dr. Chassaing told me. "Maybe you have a microbiome that is resistant to the impact of emulsifiers. Maybe I do not and am more sensitive to emulsifiers. Perhaps in several years we will be able to identify whose microbiome is more sensitive to them."[83]

For now, Dr. Chassaing's lab has completed a first of its kind clinical trial for food additives, where sixteen participants were studied in an in-patient setting and had all their meals provided to them. The participants received the same food, save for a single food additive, carboxymethylcellulose (also called cellulose gum). Quickly after starting the study, the carboxymethylcellulose-consuming participants experienced a shift toward greater inflammation-inducing organisms in their gastrointestinal tracts.

Dr. Chassaing called this a gold-standard study but one that is incredibly expensive to do. It is important to note here that not all studies are created equal. When researchers can study human beings in a controlled environment (meaning keeping all variables, save one, the same), have an intervention group and a placebo group, and look at what happens after the substance gets consumed, the results are more likely to be accurate. On the other hand, the results of surveys asking people to recall what they ate the previous year would be far more prone to error. (We don't always remember correctly, and if something bad happens, we sometimes tell people what we think they want us to say—also known as recall bias and response bias.)

But studying large groups of humans is expensive, not to mention fraught with ethical issues that require the researchers to get approval from committees meant to safeguard participants' welfare during the trial. Permission from such committees can take months or even longer. Figuring out everything that these myriad substances are doing to our guts and the rest of our bodies may take a while. In the meantime, rates of noncommunicable diseases are rising quickly, causing some in public health fields to ask for a scaling back in the consumption of ultra-processed foods based on the evidence we have today.[84] This hasn't yet happened in most industrialized nations, which are instead consuming more of them.

Based on existing research, however, there are some effects that we can pretty definitively tie to emulsifiers. By feeding, or perhaps overfeeding, part of our microbiomes while underfeeding other parts, we are causing the long-established symbiotic relationship with our intestinal residents to change. Certain additives have also been linked to inflammation. And that *is* a big deal.

Growing the Weeds, Fanning the Flames

Following the success of food gums in the 1960s and 1970s, modified food starches started gaining in popularity in the 1980s.[85] Food gums and modified starches make food smoother, able to withstand extreme temperatures (hence their popularity for use in frozen treats—no ice crystals when kept in the freezer for many months), and act as emulsifiers—keeping fat-soluble and water-soluble ingredients mixed. The term *modified starch* actually encompasses dozens of different additives, but they have certain features in common.

First, let's consider what an unmodified starch is. A starch is a complex sugar otherwise known as a carbohydrate that (normally) can be broken down into its component sugars by the body. Unmodified, naturally occurring starches are found in foods such as potatoes, rice, and wheat. Naturally occurring starches are basically just long chains of glucose that the body does not generally have trouble breaking down into simple glucose molecules that are digested quickly and easily.

When starches are modified, the chemical bonds are altered, and the body, which breaks down some bonds easily and others not so easily, does not readily break these down anymore. Instead, the body has to rely on gut bacteria to digest the modified starch.[86]

How well this happens probably differs depending on an individual's unique microbiome composition—how much of which bacteria people have in their intestines—and, as we discussed in chapter 1, this varies widely from person to person. Although animal studies have been done on the cancer-causing poten-tial of these substances (none has been found), the animals fed some modified starches were found to have increased fecal production and larger colons as a consequence of this ingestion. Some of the modified food starches used have been found to cause gastrointestinal distress in infants[87] and others have shown laxative effects in adults.[88]

Food gums and modified starches are classified by some as prebiotics, or food for the bacteria and fungi in our guts (more on this in the next chapter).[89] But it is important to remember that a side effect of bacterial digestion, or fermentation, is gas. Fermentation is just the bacteria's way of breaking down carbohydrates without the need for oxygen—producing energy for the bacteria and also differ-ent acids and gases as end products. We've known this for a really long time. It's why beer has bubbles (gas) and why sourdough bread is sour (acid). But different organisms produce different end products. For instance, wine doesn't have bub-bles unless it's sparkling or has gone off because the wrong kind of fermenting organisms got into that batch. What the bacteria are digesting, which bacteria (or fungi) are doing the digesting, and how bacteria are digesting determine if gases (and which types of gases) are produced. Digestion of food gums by gut bacteria produces a lot of gas and stool[90] and probably results in a greater likeli-hood of feeling bloated after consuming them.

I couldn't find any studies comparing the gas produced by people eating a lot of emulsifiers like food gums and modified starches to people not eating them,

When the Body Can't Break Down Sugars

The human body makes different enzymes to break down various complex sugars. But sometimes it doesn't make certain enzymes. This is how lactose intolerance occurs. For patients who suffer from lactose intolerance, the body doesn't make enough lactase enzyme to break down the milk sugar, lactose. And when that sugar passes through the gut undigested, it can bring on symptoms like gas, bloating, and diarrhea. This reaction is particularly relevant to keep in mind as we talk about what happens when the body is presented with a modified starch.

but among my patients who experience gastrointestinal problems, many note a lot of odd-smelling or bad-smelling gas when foods containing them are part of their diet. This is unsurprising. There is excellent science behind the effects that nondigestible, long-chain carbohydrates can have on our microbiome. There has been causation shown around this, and what we are feeding our microbiome matters a lot.[91]

We have put things into our food supply that are growing the weeds in our intestinal landscape. If it were just a little bit, our good bacteria, our lovely flowers, might be able to overcome the weeds. But, again, we are no longer eating just a little bit of emulsifier in an occasional snack. It is estimated that 57 percent of a typical American diet is made up of ultra-processed foods.[92]

Many ultra-processed foods contain a substance called soy lecithin. Soy lecithin (or lecithin derived from any other source) is another emulsifier meant to keep substances that would naturally separate together and smoother. It's in a lot of chocolate, nonstick cooking sprays, chips and dips, and dressings. In small amounts it probably does nothing harmful. It may even help us lubricate our stools since lecithin is a known component of the mucus that lines our guts.[93] It has also been used as a treatment for IBD.[94]

What happens when we eat larger amounts of lecithin? People taking lecithin supplements on purpose may suffer from nausea, diarrhea, and abdominal cramping.[95] Eat enough of it and you might suffer from these things, too. So how much lecithin, mostly in the form of added soy lecithin, are we eating? Odds are, for some people, it's too much.

The FDA has set no limit on the amount of lecithin that can be used in foods.[96] Though soy lecithin is used globally, we in the US tend to put it in almost every ultra-processed food.

So we are perhaps ingesting more additives than our intestinal landscape can handle, and our weeds are growing wild—so wild, in fact, that they may be breaking through our fences. And that, in turn, may fan the flames of inflammation.

When we first returned from Italy and I decided to get rid of emulsifiers and thickening agents from my diet, I enthusiastically included my husband in the project. And though it seemed that he was a willing participant, he did not enjoy taking extra time to read ingredient lists and sometimes defaulted to picking up our old staples. After a trip to the supermarket, I grabbed the cream cheese he had bought and began reciting the ingredients to him. He appeared distracted and not at all interested until I stumbled over the word "carrageenan."

"What did you say?" he asked me, finally making eye contact.

"Car-ra-gee-nan," I sounded out.

"No way!" he said and reached to inspect the container. As he read the ingredients his face fell. "I used this stuff to cause inflammation in mice when I did lab research. On purpose. We used carrageenan to cause inflammation to test treatments to cure it."

He proceeded to throw the container into the trash. Carrageenan, widely used as an emulsifier, has indeed been implicated in causing gut inflammation in both animals and humans. It still finds its way into many dairy products and dairy alternatives like soy and nut milks. The negative data around carrageenan has been accumulating for a while.[97]

Based on the evidence against carrageenan, the National Organic Standards Board voted in 2016 to remove it from foods that carry the organic label. But the US Department of Agriculture, which assigns the USDA Organic labeling for food, decided to reverse the Organic Standards Board's decision, keeping carrageenan in certified organic products.[98] The European Union (EU), however, has banned carrageenan in infant formula.[99]

Besides carrageenan, other additives such as polysorbate 80,[100] used in frostings and commercially made desserts, and carboxymethylcellulose, used as a thickening agent in a variety of foods, have been shown to induce inflammation in several studies.[101] A proposed mechanism for this is the emulsifier-induced breakdown of the lining of the gastrointestinal tract that allows for translocation, or movement, of the bacteria across the intestinal barrier, which then causes the body to react to the bacteria as if they were foreign invaders.[102] These studies have been so compelling that, as mentioned in the following box *The Case Against Emulsifiers*, several diets recommended to patients with IBD eliminate these additives entirely.

When the additive-free cream cheese isn't available at our local market, I've offered to pick up the kind with just a little bit of food gum in it because less is probably better, and perfect is the enemy of good. Plus, our kids really like cream cheese.

My husband has noticed the difference that eliminating emulsifiers from his diet has made for him, and now he's a better label reader than I am. (Also, for the record, he is very sorry for having induced inflammation in the mice.)

Now that we understand how common these ingredients can be in our food, I hope I've converted you into an enthusiastic label reader, too. Admittedly, it can be tough to avoid these foods. In the next chapter, we'll look at why.

The Case Against Emulsifiers:
Evidence from Patients with IBD

Many emulsifiers are thought to be so harmful to susceptible intestines[103] that in 2020, the IOIBD advised Crohn's disease and UC sufferers to reduce the intake of emulsifiers along with artificial sweeteners, titanium dioxide, sulfites, and trans fats.[104]

The Crohn's disease exclusion diet (CDED) eliminates the same emulsifiers, along with food gums, entirely. It was first proposed as a therapy for children with Crohn's disease who were failing to develop properly for lack of being able to eat normally. It involved an entirely liquid diet at first and then a partial liquid diet that had to be continued indefinitely. It worked, leading the researchers to ask if it might also work for adults and without the liquid diet part. In 2022, the researchers published their findings. By eating a whole-food diet, which eliminated packaged foods and bottled dressings in general and many emulsifiers and artificial sweeteners specifically, it induced clinical remission in nearly half the patients over the course of the study, which ran for twenty-four weeks.[105] It should be noted that the CDED also eliminated dairy and wheat products, fried foods, and animal fats, and was highly prescriptive in terms of what could be eaten. Adhering to the CDED necessitated working with a dietician. It was, after all, designed for patients who had an incredible amount of damage to their guts.

Diets similar to the CDED are being developed by other researchers. One of these is called the inflammatory bowel disease anti-inflammatory diet (IBD-AID) and is being developed at the University of Massachusetts. As with many of the other suggested colitis diets, IBD-AID focuses on whole foods but also emphasizes avoiding emulsifiers. It additionally encourages consuming more fermented foods. Barbara Olendzki, a registered dietician and the director of the Center for Applied Nutrition at the University of Massachusetts Chan Medical School, developed the diet and considers it a diet in evolution as we learn more and more about our gut-microbiome-environment interactions. As much as it is a diet looking toward the future, it is one that also looks back. She noted that in the 1950s our diets were different from what they are today, and that has had a huge impact on our health.

"We have a problem of not having enough and of having too much," she told me. "There are four components to IBD-AID. [We need] probiotic foods like yogurt, kefir, miso, sauerkraut. A lot of cultures have fermented foods. [We need] prebiotic foods that support the diversity of the microbiome—dark leafy greens, oats—they impact digestion. [We need] good nutrition. And we need to avoid adverse foods that contain [certain additives]."[106]

Given the severity of this disease, it makes sense that the IBD doctors and dieticians were first to move on evidence that eliminating certain additives might help their patients. But what if someone doesn't have IBD? Is it worth it to eliminate the substances that have been linked with perturbation of the microbiome and inflammation? Professor Olendzki thinks so. (She also reminded me that we have to include foods that promote a healthy microbiome, not just eliminate the bad stuff—more on probiotics in chapter 3.) Although much of her published data is on IBD, she has noted that improving what we eat can have positive effects on health in general. "Diet is related to every disease I can think of," she told me, pointing out that the diet recommended for IBD also works for the metabolic syndrome, diabetes, multiple sclerosis, rheumatoid arthritis, and IBS.

Chapter 3

Why It's Hard to Eat Real Food

*I know once people get connected to real
food, they never change back.*

—*Alice Waters*

You might already be familiar with Palm Beach, Florida. If not, it's where some of the wealthiest Americans live ensconced in multimillion-dollar beachfront estates. It is home to extravagant winter (called the season in Palm Beach speak) charity galas, which raise eight- and nine-figure donations for prominent institutions. But just over the bridge from the island of Palm Beach is the city of West Palm Beach, where 16 percent of the population lives in poverty and nearly 20 percent lacks health insurance.[107] These starkly different worlds rarely mingle—unless you happen to be in a medical office situated right between the two. I worked in one and often saw patients struggling just to get by, and patients who could buy whatever they wanted, on the same day. One winter morning, I saw two of these patients back-to-back. Their financial circumstances couldn't have been more different, and yet health-wise they had a lot in common.

Betsy was a fashionable Palm Beach socialite in her early sixties, with high blood pressure, high cholesterol, and type 2 diabetes. Her blood work was also starting to show signs of NAFLD. Owing to the season's almost nightly galas and the food that was being served, Betsy was falling short of her blood sugar goals. She felt that turning down what was being offered would be rude of her. Curious about whether we could find better choices for her, I asked her what was being

51

served at these galas. To my great shock, Betsy went on to describe a popular appetizer, which I later learned was officially known as a Palm Beach cheese puff. It is basically white bread topped with mayonnaise and cheese, then formed into a ball and baked until brown. I tried to imagine how this delicacy might not be filled with emulsifiers and ultra-processed, but I just couldn't. The rest of the food she described sounded slightly more appetizing, if not particularly whole food–based. Yes, I agreed, it would be challenging to make better choices in such an environment. And so in line with her preferences, we increased her medication instead.

Just after Betsy, I saw Valerie for her follow-up visit. Valerie, a woman in her early fifties, also struggled with type 2 diabetes, her blood pressure, cholesterol, and her blood work, too, was starting to show signs of NAFLD. But Valerie didn't attend the galas on Palm Beach. Holding down three jobs with two teenage kids at home, she rarely had time for herself. She'd grab a fast-food breakfast on the way to her first job, which started before the sun came up, and then she'd eat whatever was available for lunch on the way to her second. On the weekends, she worked her third job and didn't have much time at all for meal prep. She had been trying to spare her teenagers the burdens of housework so they could focus on school, so she didn't want to ask them to help. She wasn't sure she trusted them in the kitchen anyway. So we increased her medication, too.

These two nearly medically identical patients with drastically different circumstances still bounce around in my head despite these encounters having been years ago. While it was easier to immediately empathize with Valerie and harder to do so with Betsy, who seemed to have infinitely more choices and resources than Valerie did, I reminded myself that blaming the patient for their disease is never productive and rarely accurate. The rise of diet-related diseases at all income levels (although worse in Americans who have lower incomes)[108] is a stark reminder that something is going wrong with our food supply everywhere. Diet-related diseases are not diseases of sloth or of gluttony. Nearly all of us know someone or are someone who has had their life deeply impacted by diabetes, bowel disorders, or something that is yet to be diagnosed but is making them feel miserable. Even in Italy, where a few years ago I was able to escape ultra-processed foods for a while, recent surveys have found that a quarter of the typical Italian diet is ultra-processed.[109] Dr. Monteiro tells me that through public health interventions, Brazil has been able to slow the rise of ultra-processed food in the typical diet, but it still is over 20 percent. Recently, it was estimated that 30 percent of the average French diet is ultra-processed.[110] The US, however, has been using ultra-processed additives longer and more widely than other countries, and Americans now get the majority of their calories from ultra-processed sources.[111] Even when people are trying to eat healthfully, they may be consuming several ultra-processed or otherwise altered food products in their daily diets.

We've all heard the advice to shop the perimeter of the supermarket to avoid the less healthy foods, sticking mainly to produce, the dairy case, meats, and freshly baked breads. So perhaps you've already sworn off ranch-flavored chips and shelf-soft cookies. Noting that processed snack foods have unhealthy additives is probably not going to make the news anytime soon. Most people trying to do better with their diets are avoiding the inside aisles in the supermarket anyway. But even when shopping the perimeter, we may still wind up filling our carts with emulsifier-filled yogurts, gum-laden nondairy milks, and adulterated breads that can wreak havoc on our systems (we'll talk more about how to spot these in part II). When these potentially gut-unfriendly additives make their way into the foods that we would least suspect, it makes sticking to a gut-friendly diet tricky at best. When we make what we think are good choices (or at least better ones) and wind up feeling sick anyway, the battle with our body seems unwinnable.

Imagine a race where the finish line keeps moving. You run faster and faster and yet cannot reach the finish line no matter how hard you try. Eventually, you will give up. So many dieters and those suffering with diet-related diseases have given up. You think you are following the rules and maybe getting a little better, but then you feel awful again. You move forward but are pushed, left to guess at what might have caused the setback. Please don't blame yourself; food manufacturers are banking on us not looking too closely at the choices we're making.

Being Undone by Marketing

Like my patients, I had been avoiding foods that struck me as unhealthy, while being undone by foods that were marketed as better choices. We assume that the additives going into our foods will be okay for us to consume, particularly if that food is wrapped in packaging that calls itself organic or perhaps vegan or gluten-free. The latest term to become abused again is *clean*, perhaps indicating foods without sugar or corn syrup but potentially still containing a myriad of gut-disturbing additives. Packages that claim to be clean may still have substances like food gums or modified starches in them. Harvard Health notes that there is no accepted definition for *clean* and cautions, "In many cases, a cult-like extremism is encouraged by wellness bloggers and celebrities who have no nutrition qualifications or evidence to back up some of their promises, including claims that their version of clean eating will change your life or cure your health issues."[112] In the 150 years since *clean* was first employed to market food—breakfast cereals, as it turns out (more on that in chapter 6)[113]—the term has been reborn, but it hasn't become any more accurate.

Many granola bars and other quick energy bars marketed as being whole and healthy are essentially candy bars by another name. They are often loaded with sugar or high-fructose corn syrup, which by now most of us know to avoid, and can have added emulsifiers in them.

In the past few years, inulin, otherwise known as chicory root fiber, started to appear on labels. Inulin may also be extracted from Jerusalem artichokes, but for the purposes of the ultra-processed food industry, chicory root is used more often. Chicory root extract or fiber is a food gum equivalent. It is digested, or not, in the same way food gums are. It sounds a lot nicer though. Inulin sounds vaguely medical. Chicory root extract sounds like something you might find in your garden (or someone's garden).

That the food industry has rebranded the industrial-sounding *inulin* with the far more appetizing *chicory root extract* is at least historically consistent. In the early 1900s, *corn syrup* was considered a misleading term by the pure food activists of the day. They preferred the more chemically accurate term *glucose*, which is what it actually is (note that the more common high-fructose corn syrup used today is a combination of somewhat more troublesome fructose and glucose sugars, while unadulterated corn syrup is just glucose sugar molecules). The food processors felt that the word *glucose* was too much like the word *glue* and off-putting for consumers. They were able to convince government regulators of that, and the more pleasant term *corn syrup* was born.[114]

By using terms that describe what these ingredients are derived from, food producers argue that they are being even more transparent, informing consumers where their products are coming from. If that isn't convincing enough, there has been a recent push to mount scientific evidence in favor of adding inulin, or chicory root extract, to food for health reasons—and many scientists and physicians are jumping on board.

Inulin is a soluble, fermentable fiber—basically ideal food for some bacterial species in our microbiomes. Studies have shown that taking inulin increases the frequency of defecation for those with constipation.[115] Is inulin a beneficial additive? For some, it may be—or it might not. More on this in chapter 7. Our microbiomes are so varied that what may be helpful for one person just may not be for another. There isn't going to be a one-size-fits-all approach here. But we should approach any health claims about food additives with a healthy amount of skepticism.

At present, it is unclear to what extent different bacterial species might be promoted or inhibited by the various nondigestible substances that are used as emulsifiers and thickeners in our food. Are we growing flowers or weeds with the additive fertilizers we are putting into our gastrointestinal gardens? What seems to be going on in the guts of diet-related disease sufferers is that the weeds are being promoted over the flowers and overgrowing in places where they are not wanted.

When it applies to digestion, eating an ultra-processed food item with an additive derived from a natural source mixed into it is not the same as consuming the whole food the additive comes from.

A 2016 study showed that purified prebiotic fibers similar to inulin did not help heal the intestines of mice who had been deprived of natural fiber-rich foods.[116] Yet another study showed a substantially increased risk of liver cancer in mice who were receiving inulin supplementation in an effort to improve their blood sugar. Importantly, this was not designed as a cancer study. The researchers were looking for the inulin to do something beneficial for the mice and were seemingly pro-inulin. But surprisingly, they found that it produced cancer in their test subjects. In their paper, they advise that "enriching foods with fiber to manipulate microbiota should be approached with great caution."[117] However, research is indeed emerging that whole, intact chicory root increases the diversity of gut microbiomes, and there is reasonable evidence to consider that having more and different bacteria is better.[118]

The Probiotic Problem

We can't talk about marketing, health, and the microbiome without talking about the probiotic industry. It is thought that having a predominance of helpful bacteria in our microbiome may lead to better physical and mental health. So why not ingest some of the species known to be beneficial? Enter probiotics. A probiotic is a supplement that contains actual gut bacteria, usually some combination of bifidobacteria and lactobacilli with a few others sometimes thrown in for good measure.

Today, fixing our intestines has become a multibillion-dollar industry. Americans spent an estimated $2 billion on probiotic supplements in 2017, which had doubled since just five years earlier.[119] While probiotics sound promising, there is little evidence for how best to deliver them to the gut or which ones in which proportions are actually the right combination of beneficial bacteria. How many of these bacteria survive the trip through the acidic environment of the stomach to set up shop in our intestines is hotly debated. Probiotics may help with antibiotic-induced diarrhea, but the science around the rest is shaky. Basically, we don't yet know which bacteria to consume, in what quantities, or how often. It isn't clear that many of these bacteria survive the drugstore shelf, let alone the journey through our gastrointestinal system to take up any sort of permanent residence in our microbiomes. And the vast majority of supplements on the supermarket or vitamin store shelf also contain the very additives that may be supporting a maladapted microbiome in the first place.

To avoid capsules and embrace real food, some people have joined the feeding frenzy around fermented foods, which are also probiotics—meaning they contain bacteria and sometimes yeast and prebiotics, which is the food that nourishes the probiotics. And while there isn't definitive evidence yet, a 2021 study lends support to the idea that if it's not quite right to choose fermentation over fiber (which we definitely need lots of from whole foods), then eating fermented foods as an addition to our diets is a reasonable alternative to pills.[120]

Two groups of patients were studied—one group was told to eat a great deal more fiber, and the other was instructed to eat more fermented food like yogurt and kombucha. The folks in the fiber arm of the study noted softer stools. The fermented-food eaters experienced some initial bloating, which resolved in a few weeks, signifying that something was changing in their guts.

The researchers tested the participants' stools throughout the study to find out just what was happening. The fiber-eaters' stools showed an increase in the amount of bacteria that favor fiber's carbohydrate fuel, but the type of bacteria that flourished in each person tended to be the bacteria they already had. They now just had more of them.

In contrast, the fermented-food eaters' stool didn't show more bacteria, but rather different bacteria—intriguingly not necessarily the bacteria that was in the fermented food itself. Somehow, the fermented-food participants' microbiomes were changing and acquiring additional bacterial species from somewhere. Had they been hiding out deep in the colonic crypts? Maybe. Were they friend or foe? They were possibly good friends whom we had lost touch with for far too long. Why were they most likely friendly? Well, the researchers also monitored the subjects' blood for inflammatory markers that are sometimes harbingers of disease, and the markers had decreased in the fermented-food group, perhaps heralding better health.

So should we run out and buy so-called living food—stocking up on kefir and sauerkraut? If you like that sort of thing, sure. But the main takeaway from this remarkable study is that what we eat can manipulate our microbiomes in a much more impactful way than taking a pill might. That is incredibly empowering but also a little bit worrisome. It means we need to start paying attention to what exactly we are feeding the little creatures in our guts.

There appears to be a difference, a big difference, between intact foods and ultra-processed foods that have had individual components taken out of intact foods and then inserted into the ultra-processed ones. The data for any one treatment or additive is usually not terribly strong, but we are experiencing an avalanche of evidence telling us to eat mostly whole foods[121] and avoid the ultra-processed stuff when possible. It's important to remember that, at least for now, the burden of avoiding these foods is on us. In most cases, we can't rely on our regulatory agencies to catch up to the science and enact policies to protect us. Let's look at the example of trans fats to see why.

Holding Out for a Hero? (Why We Can't Wait for a Ban)

Partially hydrogenated oils are liquid fats that have been turned solid in the lab by altering some chemical bonds. They are then called *trans fats*. Since trans fats exist in some foods, where they naturally occur in small amounts, they were long thought to be safe. Recall that we base a lot of our ideas about food safety on the principle that if it exists in whole foods, we should be able to safely extract it or create it in the lab and add it to our ultra-processed items. So, hydrogenated oils, starting out as a liquid extracted from plants and then chemically altered or "hydrogenated" to become solid, were thought to be an improvement on animal fats like butter. Trans fats keep foods shelf-stable for a long time and were thus added to many highly processed food items for decades before evidence began to mount against them.

About eighty years after trans fats were introduced, studies in the 1990s started linking foods with added trans fats to heart disease. And this time, the data was unequivocal. It was estimated that by banning trans fats, we would prevent twenty thousand heart attacks and seven thousand deaths in the US a year, leading the FDA in 2018 to ban the largest source of trans fats—the partially hydrogenated oils.[122] (As a side note, trans fats have also been implicated in causing changes to the gut mucosa and possibly being related to irritable bowel symptoms.[123] So avoiding trans fats for gastrointestinal reasons, as well as cardiovascular health, is probably a good idea.)

Interestingly, the use of mono- and diglycerides has risen in the wake of the trans fat ban since they are also fats and can perform a lot of the same functions that the partially hydrogenated oils used to. They are ubiquitous in ultra-processed foods, and it is argued that we are only eating small amounts of them (though that probably depends on the quantity of packaged foods one eats). Their effect on our cardiovascular system and our bowels have not been studied very much yet. Given the gastrointestinal relief patients seem to have when avoiding these additives, getting rid of mono- and diglycerides from our diets seems like a reasonable thing to do. However, the FDA hasn't banned them yet and may never do so since the evidence required for a ban needs to be overwhelming and, as with trans fats, could take decades to amass. Also, recall the issues with studies on additives that I pointed out in the previous chapter:

- Studies are often funded by biased parties
- Studies are often small
- Research looks at compounds in isolation, not as combinations
- Studies in animals are often intriguing but are not guaranteed to hold true for humans
- Research on humans is incredibly expensive to do

The stringency of FDA regulations has waxed and waned over the years, and we now appear to be in a waning period. Perhaps, then, we could turn to our brethren across the Atlantic to guide us through the morass of food additives?

In 2015, the EFSA created a list of 316 food additives that they intended to re-evaluate. As of the writing of this book, 112 additives still remain to be re-evaluated, including carrageenan, mono- and diglycerides, cellulose gum (also called carboxymethylcellulose), xanthan gum, locust bean gum, and lecithins. The call for data to be submitted around most of these additives was supposed to remain open into 2020 and was started to address the data gaps that were found in the previous scientific opinions by the group.[124] Due to the coronavirus pandemic, the deadline for the data is now mid-2022. It is important to note that nearly half the members of the EFSA have financial ties to the food industry—with a quarter receiving direct payments from the industry and many more belonging to organizations that take money from food businesses.[125] While incredibly commonplace in academia in the US, Europe is certainly not immune to influence, either. The interests of industry influences regulation of food additives everywhere.[126]

Indeed, many food additives that have been approved around the world, not just in the US, have gotten that approval with little scientific evidence. Very few human studies have been done for most additives, and those have generally been done on just a few healthy young participants being fed the additive for short periods of time. Children are almost never studied, and very young children and infants are only studied to prove that an additive is not obviously and immediately harmful, not that it is innocuous and should be in our food supply.

In the US, there hasn't been an outcry from the scientific community on the paucity of evidence, but, rather, the professional low rumble about the lack of standards has fallen to the free trade enthusiasts and lawyers. It turns out that the more stringent EU rules currently in existence, and the potential for more stringent EU rules in the near future, have engaged the lawyers who will be expected to navigate the trade rules between the US and EU.[127]

Yet the global food additive industry is worth the equivalent of the economic output of some small countries, and it's possible that the European Commission charged with formulating the usage guidelines for food additives will give them the benefit of the doubt where doubt remains. It also remains to be seen whether these regulations will make it to the US. As Tim Lang and Erik Millstone write in the *Lancet*, a well-regarded UK-based medical journal, "when European expert advisors reach different conclusions, it is not because they fail to accept the evidence; rather, they ask and answer different questions and consequently look at different bodies of evidence" than advisors do in the US.[128] We are therefore left to try to sort through the less than ideal evidence that exists on the ingredients in our food and make our own decisions about what we want to consume.

Everything Is Processed?

Dr. Monteiro told me a story to illustrate the insidious rise of ultra-processed food in Brazil. He was aghast to see that highly processed foods were being marketed to an increasingly younger audience and recounted how a highly refined starch pressed into starlike shapes that would dissolve quickly in the mouth was being marketed to children just learning to self-feed.

"Babies less than one year old!" he declared, incredulous that children too young to walk or talk were being enticed by ultra-processed food items.

It did seem shocking. Until I realized that I knew exactly the product he was referring to.

"We call those puffs in the US," I told him, recalling how I would drop a handful onto the tray on my children's stroller to keep them quiet and occupied as I ran my errands.

Yes, he agreed. That would be a rough translation of what was being marketed in Brazil. He went on to tell me how he had tried to fight to keep the Brazilian puffs out of the food supply or to at least limit the marketing—all to no avail. I might have audibly sighed. These had been a normal pantry item in my house. As a young mother I loved anything that kept the kids occupied for any length of time. But these were not normal to Dr. Monteiro, who was seeing them for the first time. These were novel food-like items being pushed on Brazilian babies with potential implications for what they thought of as good snack foods later in life.

If we have to resort to an ultra-processed product, we can select the one with the least amount of potentially gut-roiling additives. This does make a difference—one that we've mostly been asked to ignore. Maybe you've heard that nearly everything is processed and have given up on trying to sort the good processing out from the bad (or the good merely processed versus the bad ultra-processed, according to the Nova classification system). That's to be expected. There's been a lot of money spent by the food industry to get you, as well as doctors and dieticians, to think this way.

In her book, *Unsavory Truth*, nutrition professor Marion Nestle outlines how multinational food companies that manufacture ultra-processed foods try to paint themselves in the best possible light by sometimes funding or applying other sources of pressure on dieticians, researchers, and even journalists.[129] Often this means obscuring just what an ultra-processed food is. The next time you see a post on social media by someone with letters after their name telling you that it is impossible to tell what is or isn't an ultra-processed food, consider that they may have been influenced by "big food."

Slow progress, however, is being made. In November of 2021, the American Heart Association finally cautioned people to "choose minimally processed foods instead of ultra-processed foods" in their guidelines but included the caveat that "there is no commonly accepted definition for ultra-processed foods, and some healthy foods may exist within the ultra-processed food category."[130] This caveat is slightly misleading, however.

Researchers have indeed come up with a handy, if not particularly brief, definition of an ultra-processed foods. They are "industrial formulations which, besides salt, sugar, oils and fats, include substances not used in culinary preparations, in particular additives used to imitate sensorial qualities of minimally processed foods and their culinary preparations."[131] In other words, they are the food products that use the emulsifiers and thickeners (along with other categories of additives) that have been implicated in diet-related diseases. It is to the great advantage of the food industry to make you believe that all food is processed, and there's no way to begin to untangle the mess of ultra-processed food infiltration into your life. But we can walk this trend back. When we choose a product with fewer or no emulsifiers, thickeners, or stabilizers, we are indeed making a healthier choice and sending a message to food manufacturers that they need to begin to scale back the level of processing in their products. Unfortunately, this isn't a choice all of us can make.

The Poor Carry More Than Their Share of the Burden

Those one-dollar snack cakes may be an indulgence for the middle-class shopper who tosses them into her shiny shopping cart in her neighborhood's brightly lit and well-stocked supermarket. On the other hand, they may be breakfast for the barely-getting-by day laborer who picks them up at the convenience store on her way to a job when the person giving her a ride stops to get gas. More than 5 percent of Americans live in what have been labeled food deserts—places where little more than ultra-processed food is generally available and where finding affordable, nutritious whole foods is nearly impossible.[132]

It is impractical to suggest that everyone can easily give up cheap ultra-processed foods. But the impact that being dependent on ultra-processed foods is having on our health is becoming an increasingly important public health issue. And when you are poor, health issues have many times the impact on your life compared to those who have the financial resources to be able to take time off work for medical appointments and sick days, as well as have insurance to help pay for medications. Many agricultural workers have no access to toilet facilities during the day, making the burden of an irritable bowel or the ability to inject insulin in a clean environment incredibly complicated. Medications for diabetes can run into thousands of dollars per month without insurance (and even hundreds with insurance). Not being able to avoid ultra-processed foods has much more of an impact on those living in impoverished neighborhoods, disproportionately communities of color in the US, than on those for whom these food are a choice. We are all eating way too much ultra-processed food, especially ultra-processed snacks. But for some of us, there aren't readily available or affordable alternatives.

I want to make it clear that I'm not criticizing anyone for what they have to do to feed their families or get some enjoyment out of life. We have a long way to go to get healthier foods into everyone's hands. But many of us can make changes—and they don't have to be expensive or difficult. That's what we'll talk about in the next chapter and the following two parts of this book.

Chapter 4

How to Eat an Elephant

How do you eat an elephant?
One bite at a time.

—Proverb

Eating ultra-processed foods has become a way of life for so many of us. If it wasn't part of our culture twenty, thirty, or seventy years ago, it almost certainly is now, wherever in the world we might find ourselves. With approximately half of the foods we eat containing these additives and the additives sometimes going by healthy-sounding names, you may be asking how you can eat anything, let alone everything. If we define "everything" as all foods without gut-roiling additives, things that our grandparents or perhaps great-grandparents would have recognized as food, or "real food" if you will, we can indeed eat everything. And the good news is that real food is still out there. You just have to know where to find it.

Dr. Monteiro says it is not hard to go from an ultra-processed food to a less processed one. And Professor Olendzki tells me that it is easier to eliminate foods from one's diet than to add them. So how do we start to change our diets? Well, I propose we start with one bite— or, rather, not taking some bites. We are not going to start eating a raw or vegan diet (unless you are already doing this, which is fine, but probably not an attainable goal for most). But we can do a lot of healing and promote good health by starting with the biggest elephant in the nutrition room—getting rid of the additives that are doing none of us any good and are possibly doing a great deal of harm to some of us.

Eliminating emulsifiers and other additives that disrupt the microbiome is a great first step—in fact, it's a giant leap—in the right direction. It might be the only one you take, and that's just fine. It's actually fantastic. You may also want to follow a more prescriptive eating plan for your specific health concern or for environmental or moral reasons. Unless you have to avoid a specific food item due to your personal health history, eat whatever you like that's real food.

As you start your journey to ditching emulsifiers, you may want to take one (or all!) of these three steps: eat like your ancestors (or someone's), get back to the kitchen, and reclaim the joy of food.

Eat Like Your Ancestors, or Someone's

Italians, of course, don't have a monopoly on healthy eating. Though the Mediterranean diet has been lauded for its heart healthiness and my own Italian experiment has indicated its gut friendliness, there are other diets from Africa, Asia, and Latin America that may be just as beneficial. These traditional diets have scratch cooking and nutrient-dense ingredients as their hallmarks, and it turns out that all so-called heritage diets may support a healthy microbiome.[133]

So, yes, eat like an Italian if you like that sort of thing. Or don't, if you prefer something else. If traditional African or Asian or Latin American foods are more appealing, eat those. Traditional, regional US cuisine is great, too. Heavily influenced by African American, Native American, and Latin American recipes, Cajun, New England, and Southwestern food should not be overlooked. If all we consider are hamburgers and fries when we think of American food, we are missing out. But what you eat may need to hew more closely to the foods that your grandparents or great-grandparents ate, because the foods that your parents are eating are probably too ultra-processed. If you no longer have an older, tradition-based adult to consult, organizations are springing up to help guide eager eaters through the world of their forebears.

Oldways is a Boston-based nutritional not-for-profit organization offering traditional recipes along five pathways—Mediterranean, African, Asian, Latin

American, and vegetarian and vegan. They aren't trying to argue that one culture's diet is better than another's or that certain staple foods are better than others. Their thesis is that getting back to your dietary roots, or anyone's dietary roots, is a big step to better health.

Sara Baer-Sinnott, president of Oldways, explained how the organization decided on its five pathways: "We are a nation of many cultures and one size doesn't fit all." Oldways was created to honor food traditions that were being erased across the globe in the 1980s. It was developed in an effort to bring food enthusiasts, chefs, and scientists together to help fix what seemed to be going awry with food. We wanted to bring everyone together. Not just scientists talking to scientists and chefs talking to chefs."[134]

Oldways attempts to bring everyone to the metaphorical table to figure out how to make healthy food affordable and appealing to people from a variety of food traditions. Baer-Sinnott also made it a point to explain that the five pathways are incredibly large categories but there is commonality within each pathway and across traditional eating as a whole.

"The way people in India eat is very different than the way people in China eat. But the pattern is the same."[135]

According to Baer-Sinnott, staple foods are like a chain linking various cultural traditions, with each culture putting its own spin on the cuisine. While ingredients like whole grains, tomatoes, and olive oil link various food traditions in the Mediterranean, other grains, vegetables, and spices define different regions across the globe. No matter your personal preferences, choices for delicious and healthy food abound. It's just a matter of learning from tradition and getting back to whole ingredients.

What, exactly, is a whole ingredient? Ideally, it is an ingredient that looks as close to its starting point as possible. If it looks the same as it did when it was harvested, it is a whole ingredient. While eating just whole ingredients is ideal, it isn't terribly practical for most of us. So, whenever you have the opportunity, choose less processed over more highly processed foods. And, of course, read labels when shopping for the ingredients you are going to use. If you are using pre-shredded cheese or supermarket bread, make sure the additives aren't in there.

But wait. How can this be a book about eating everything if I keep telling you to avoid foods with additives, particularly those emulsifiers and thickeners?

By *eat everything* I mean that you can eat everything that is meant to be eaten. No one would suggest eating banana leaves (though they are natural and make fun food wrappers) or the plastic wheels on a toy car (though children have tried). These are simply not meant to be eaten. So, no, if we are being linguistic purists, you cannot actually eat everything. But you can eat all the real foods that our ancestors have been eating for hundreds of years. And by *our*, I mean humankind. While your direct ancestors may not have eaten barley or quinoa or kale, many humans have ancestors who have.

Get Back to the Kitchen

As a component of ancestral diets, Baer-Sinnott also mentions that cooking at home is important. And here is where a lot of us fall down a bit—or a lot.

A *Harvard Business Review* article reported in 2017 that only 10 percent of Americans said they love to cook, down from 15 percent just fifteen years earlier.[136] Well, it's hard to love something that we aren't sure how to do, that we may not be very good at due to lack of practice, and that is, on its face, challenging. None of this sounds very fun at all.

In any change process, we must set ourselves up for success. Unless you are already an experienced cook (perhaps you are in that 10 percent who love to cook), buying complicated cookbooks or googling long internet recipes is setting yourself up for failure. But getting back to cooking doesn't have to mean you are churning out elaborate dishes for every meal. I promise it can be easy.

If you have a friend who can cook, ask for help (those 10 percenters are out there!). It's amazing how much we can learn from watching someone who knows the right temperature to heat a pan to before adding ingredients, or what *salt to taste* actually means. If you don't count a 10 percenter among your friends, that's okay, too. Find basic cookbooks that can help. I particularly enjoy cookbooks by practical home cooks—they get me. I picked up Katie Workman's *The Mom 100 Cookbook* at a school book fair when my oldest kid was in elementary school. I'm still reaching for it now that he's in high school. The recipes are pretty easy, and we usually have the ingredients on hand. And when we were overstuffed from a delicious lunch in Italy, my husband impulse-bought *A Family Farm in Tuscany* by Sarah Fioroni. Sarah is an accomplished cook and runs her family's farm-to-table establishment. Some of the recipes are a bit more challenging, but there are plenty of simple ones (I adapted one in the recipes section of this book).

Following an intricate recipe is about as challenging for me as if I were trying to perform an appendectomy by only using a textbook. I have seen a few and can appreciate a surgery done well, but far be it from me to do a complex operation unsupervised with only written instructions. I'm not a surgeon, nor am I a chef.

But making simple dishes once you get the hang of it can be a lot of fun. Turning out a good chili or pasta dish that my kids love and say that I make better than the restaurants brings me joy (so does eating it). These dishes are now staples in my house. They are easy for me to make because making them has become habitual (and chili in a slow cooker is arguably one of the easiest things for anyone to make). The first time I made these dishes, however, they were not good, and my kitchen was a mess. The second time, they were better. Now they are my signature dishes and friends ask for the recipes all the time. Practice may not make perfect, but it does make things easier. And spending a few weeks forming healthier habits has benefits that can pay off for years, and maybe even generations if our kids learn them, too.

Reclaim the Joy of Eating

Finally, let's give ourselves some grace and acknowledge that change can be challenging. It's all about getting through the transition while you form new ways of doing things. In that vein, I propose keeping the following in mind:

Don't let the perfect be the enemy of the good.
Life is hard enough, let's not make it harder.
Have fun.

This is what I tell my patients when they're trying to make lifestyle changes, and it is even more important when thinking about making dietary changes.

A Sample Weekly Plan

Are you curious about how to make cooking from home work for you? Check out appendix B of this book, where I offer a sample weekly plan for fitting in some scratch cooking as painlessly as possible.

Don't Let the Perfect Be the Enemy of the Good

While writing this book, I started to think about food more than I ever wanted to. Some days, I found myself getting downright obsessive. When that happened, I remembered that we have forgotten how to worry less about what we are eating and *just enjoy it*.

Food has become just another thing to worry about. If our intestines are calm and quiet, if our lab values are lovely but our minds are racing about what we can or can't eat from the moment we wake up, we haven't solved much.

A physician, with whom I had the great privilege of training, had a question he would ask all of his patients before discussing their illnesses. He'd ask, "What brings you joy?" This physician, as a young trainee, immediately recognized that this was the most important question you could ask a person. I started to ask patients this question, too. And after family and friends, food or eating was perhaps the most common answer. This book is intended to restore the joy of eating to people who have begun to fear it. It isn't intended to replace one fear with another.

Most diet plans are about sticking to a strict list of dos and don'ts, and most people ultimately give up on any given plan because it becomes too difficult to sustain the level of commitment needed to adhere to the plan. So we must give ourselves some grace to go off track from time to time. Some days it's just too difficult to meal plan. Some days it is just too difficult to even pick up a meal. Because sometimes jobs get too demanding, kids get sick, or we are just too exhausted. Trying to eat right takes a lot of mental energy, and some days there just isn't enough to go around. And it's okay.

Sometimes we need to just eat. So do it. Tomorrow, you can go back to avoiding ingredients that cause you GI distress, and your bowels will bounce right back. Your labs can normalize again. Humans are resilient. (Remember, your microbiome changes a lot in twenty-four hours based on what you happened to eat that day!) And unless and until it becomes a lot easier to avoid the ingredients that can upset our systems, we have to leave room to just throw up our hands some days.

Life Is Hard Enough, Let's Not Make It Harder

For something to become a habit, it has to be easy (relatively) for us to do, and we have to get some kind of psychological or physical reward for doing it. Once the behavior becomes habitual, we don't even have to think before doing it.[137] If our refrigerators and pantries are stocked with foods that are good for us, we will reach for those foods. If they are stocked with foods that are not good for us, that's what we will eat. So make it easy for yourself by doing a little planning in advance. Buy whole ingredients that you know you will use. Read ingredient lists and buy the foods with no (or fewer) additives.

Soon, you will become used to eating the good stuff and will find new foods that make you feel satisfied—without the pain. Eat a home-baked cake instead of an ultra-processed grocery one. You'll feel good, and soon enough the overly sweet, brightly colored cake doesn't look as appealing anymore. Ultra-flavored chips will no longer have the pull they once did. When you start to make better choices on a regular basis, it becomes easier and more enjoyable to do so.

Have Fun

Ask yourself what makes food fun. Is it the bright colors of the sprinkles from your childhood? The throwback bottle filled with a drink that you enjoyed with a beloved family member? The initial joy of the sprinkles and sodas come from being associated with celebrations—birthdays and team wins, making honor roll and graduation—and depending on which foods you were raised with, a savory biryani (complex rice dish) or flaky pastelitos (pastries filled with meat or guava) might do the same. Evoking memories of childhood can be powerful. A whiff of a familiar food can bring a smile to our faces before we even bring that food to our lips. (Although, if we were born in the United States anywhere from the 1950s to the modern day, the food we ate as children began to look less like actual food as our childhoods progressed. The food we are currently feeding our own children is beginning to establish memories in their minds and will be the stuff that potentially brings them joy in later years.)

The brightness and sweetness of food can be perceived as fun and evocative of joy. And, let's face it, it is. So how do we create that same level of excitement around real food? Fruit can be bright and sweet. Blend frozen dragon fruit with bananas and strawberries, and you'll get an electric pink smoothie bowl you can top with even more brightly colored fruits. This truly makes everyone happy in my house. If fruit just isn't going to do it for you, make a quick baked treat.

When we cook or bake for ourselves, we (hopefully) aren't using emulsifiers, and we tend to use less sugar than ultra-processed food purveyors do. I guarantee joy with freshly baked cookies. If the thought of the sink full of dishes I've just suggested you create is not bringing you any joy whatsoever, consider buying treats with fewer or no additives. There will be more suggestions to come in the chapters ahead, but the main idea is to start making new memories and positive associations with real food when we can. Real food can be just as enjoyable as the ultra-processed stuff we've gotten used to. Learning where we can rediscover that joy is the key to healing what ails us.

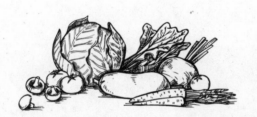

Part II

How to Eat Everything

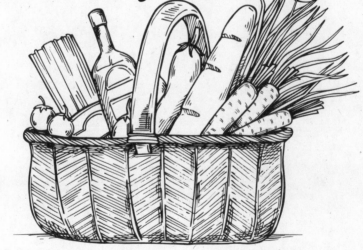

Chapter 5

Dairy

How can anyone govern a nation that has two hundred and forty-six different kinds of cheese?

—Charles de Gaulle

William, a young man in his twenties, came to me with a strange story about eating cheese. He had discovered that he felt a lot better when avoiding dairy. Not drinking milk was easy enough, but when he ate foods containing cheese—pizza or burritos—he would have to run to the bathroom with diarrhea. But through trial and error (a lot of error), he had learned that he could eat fresh mozzarella cheese.

William had read about lactose intolerance and thought he had it. Though some adults lose the ability to produce lactase, the enzyme that splits the milk sugar lactose into its more digestible components, most children have no problem digesting milk. Not so for William. He noted that his troubles with dairy had started well before he reached adulthood. He'd take the over-the-counter lactase enzyme with mixed results, and he assumed that the effectiveness or not of the pills must have to do with how much lactose the food item contained. After a while, he lost faith in the lactase-containing pills and just tried to avoid dairy foods altogether. Except for fresh mozzarella.

"Fresh mozzarella must have less lactose in it than other cheeses," he had (incorrectly) surmised.

Dairy has become quite controversial these past few years. Once thought to be an absolutely necessary dietary component—generations of children were encouraged to drink three glasses of milk daily—it's become something of a dietary villain of late. The truth, however, is probably somewhere in between—it's neither absolutely necessary nor evil.

Dairy is an important part of many cultural traditions and doesn't appear at all in others. Some people have no trouble digesting dairy products into old age, and others cannot digest it at all. Since vegans, adherents to the Paleo diet, and many others are avoiding dairy products, we've seen the rise of alternative milks made from soy, oats, and nuts—which often contain myriad gut-roiling additives. Many people don't feel any better using these products, either.

The Additives That Keep Shredded Cheese Separated

The making of fresh mozzarella could easily be ranked among the artistic wonders of Italy. On a farm tour, I watched a ropy-armed man leaning over a large metal vat transform heated milk by pulling it into cheese in a matter of minutes using what could only be described as magic. The result was warm and soft and the very definition of a comfort food. And while it had less lactose than the whole milk the cheese maker had started with, it still contained a significant amount. Certainly, it had more than a hard cheese would. Harder cheeses have less lactose since the liquid portion is the lactose-containing part of the cheese. And there should be less lactose in the firmer shredded mozzarella than in the more liquid fresh kind that William was able to enjoy.[138]

Was William sure that he had less trouble with the fresh mozzarella than the shredded kind? If it were just his lactose intolerance, it should have been the other way around. So if it wasn't the lactose that was bothering William, what was it? By now you can probably guess that I suspected additives were playing a role.

If you shred a block of hard cheese, then put it into a plastic baggie or some other kind of storage container and throw it into the fridge, within a day or two the cheese will start to clump and get stuck together. The natural moisture in the cheese will cause the clumping to occur. But the pre-shredded cheese you buy or that many restaurants use won't have that problem. The individual shreds of cheese will stay nicely separated for weeks or even months. The reason for this is that the shreds have been coated with potato starch and cellulose, a nondigestible, unfermentable fiber.

Unlike the food additives discussed earlier, which can be fermented by bacteria and encourage growth of different types of intestinal bacteria, cellulose is not considered food by bacteria. However, cellulose, an added nondigestible fiber, causes the bowels to increase motility—basically it makes the bowels speed up. This is something that might be of benefit to a constipated person but not particularly helpful to someone who already has loose stools. Additionally, it turns out that cellulose, by virtue of changing the speed of the bowels, can alter the gut's environment for the bacteria it houses—favoring the growth of species of bacteria that can further alter our intestines.[139]

Grated Parmesan cheese has been noted to be full of cellulose, with some popular brands being nearly 10 percent cellulose.[140] Parmesan is a hard cheese with little naturally occurring lactose. But grated prepackaged Parmesan cheese can be difficult for some people to digest. It's not the lactose for many. There's really only a little of that in this very hard cheese. It's the other non-cheese stuff that finds its way into our conveniently packaged products that causes the cheese troubles for many.

Sharp-eyed readers will note that cellulose does occur naturally in plants. The difference is that in plant matter it creates complex wall structures and mixes in with other fibers and substances as the naturally occurring cellulose travels through the gastrointestinal system. I am not advocating avoiding naturally occurring cellulose contained within fruits and vegetables. Please eat this. Eat lots of it. Just avoid it as an additive, where it is digested differently.

Shredded cheese also often has other preservatives because while a block of hard cheese can last a long time even when opened, shredded cheese will not. Natamycin, an antifungal agent, is often used to retard fungal growth on shredded cheese. Antibiotic and antifungal resistance is on the rise, reaching scary levels in some places, and there is fear that natamycin could be a contributing factor.[141]

This might be a good time to recall that the microbiome isn't just about bacteria, though those are the components of the microbiome that we focus on in this book. Fungi make up a smaller part of our microbiome that's even more poorly understood than the bacterial component, giving us yet another good reason to avoid pre-shredded cheese and the antifungal agents it sometimes contains.

Our time is precious, but shredding or grating cheese is pretty quick once you get the hang of it. Adding a minute or two to food prep (or asking restaurants to leave the cheese off a dish if it is the pre-shredded kind—which it almost always is) was worth it for William to be able to enjoy cheeses again.

I suggested he try hard cheese in blocks without additives and shred or slice it himself. They didn't seem to bother him—just like the fresh mozzarella! While William could now eat small amounts of hard block cheeses he shredded himself, soft cheeses were still out. His body was processing not-too-large amounts of lactose just fine. Did he continue to have to avoid soft cheeses because they contained more lactose? Maybe. But some soft cheeses and cheese spreads, cream cheese in particular, often resemble store-bought ice creams more than cheeses when the ingredient list is examined. There is heavy use of food gums and other emulsifiers in many soft cheeses to prevent the ingredients from separating, which may be the underlying problem for many of us.

Discovering Real Yogurt

One day when we were in Rome, my family and I wandered into a small co-op market for a light lunch. My daughter picked out a peach yogurt. We sat on some benches to enjoy our food, and she peeled back the foil top of her yogurt. It was unmixed and she was unsure, making a horrified face. I reassured her, noted that we try new things when traveling, and then stirred it for her. She wanted me to taste it to make sure it was okay. It was more than okay. The yogurt was smooth, creamy, and delicious. It was made with only the most basic ingredients and wasn't too sweet. A smile spread across my face, and my daughter immediately intuited that the yogurt was good. She demanded her yogurt back, and I handed it over. She took a bite and smiled too, nodding in agreement. It was good! I asked her for another bite. She playfully brought the spoon to my mouth and then pulled it away at the last second. Though often willing to share any food item, she was now adamant—the amazing yogurt was hers.

The Fungus Among Us Matter, Too

Our *myco*biome, or the fungus that makes up a small but significant component of our microbiomes, has been gaining more attention recently. Because fungus can be harder to grow in a lab than bacteria is, it wasn't until molecular methods became cheaper and easier to perform in the last few years that many of the species of fungi cohabitating with us were discovered.[142] And just like our bacteria, fungi can be either friend or foe depending on where they grow and how much they proliferate. Blasting our guts with antifungals (if the fungi aren't causing us problems), just like cavalierly destroying many bacterial species with antibiotics, probably isn't a great idea given the emerging evidence that there is overgrowth of some fungal species and a paucity of other species in certain diseases.[143]

The same ingredients that go into cream cheese also create yogurt, except that different cultures are used and sugar may be substituted for salt. In the US, yogurt is often adulterated in a fashion similar to cream cheese, by adding stabilizers and emulsifiers. In general, though, some plain yogurts available on grocery shelves in the US are often just milk or cream and cultures.

So now I buy plain Greek yogurt made only with milk and yogurt cultures and add simple ingredients like berries and nuts to it. Traditionally, Greek yogurt is made thicker by a straining process, so thickening agents aren't usually used, unlike some other popular commercially-made yogurts. Sometimes I add a little honey or maple syrup. I now stare at the myriad of yogurt choices on the grocery shelf and am not moved by any of them. I have tasted what real yogurt should be, separated and all, and I cannot go back.

I Scream, You Scream, a Lot of Us Scream After Eating Ice Cream

Before I visited Italy, I hadn't yet considered that food gums and modified food starches could be the cause of my symptoms. People with IBS are used to hearing that we have to give up all kinds of foods. The truth is that we can start to feel better when we do, encouraging us to give up more and more. This creates a bland, only marginally effective diet for ourselves and sometimes results in the extreme restrictions Emma struggled with. Before I ever considered giving up bread or gluten I, like many of my patients, thought that dairy and the lactose it contained was the cause of my bowel travails. I could easily abandon milk and more reluctantly part with cheese, but giving up ice cream represented a rejection of fun, a renunciation of childhood, and a reluctant acceptance of middle age. In other words, I didn't want to do it. But I had to. I found that eating ice cream was just about the worst thing I could do for my GI system. I thought that I was going to have to permanently part ways with one of life's most delicious indulgences. But then I picked up a spoon and tasted a bit of my kid's gelato in Italy and began to doubt a lot of what I had been doing.

The first thing I noticed was that the gelato felt different in my mouth. There was no slimy film left behind after taking a bite, which turned out to be because there were no odd remnants of stabilizing agents or emulsifiers left behind on my tongue. The other thing I noticed was that the gelato started to quickly drip down the sides of the paper cup (like the good, attentive mother that I am, I swiftly rescued these bits with my spoon). The gelato tasted much better but was also a lot messier than the ice cream we get in the US. It was melting fast in the heat—the way I remembered ice cream used to when I was a kid. We needed to use many more napkins when eating gelato in Italy (as good as the ice cream is, the napkins are terrible). Sure it was hot (hence, all the gelato), but I'm a Floridian. I do a lot of hot weather. The melting wasn't just about the heat.

An absentminded uncle once left a carton of ice cream out on the counter overnight. When I opened it the next morning, it looked only half melted. The semisolid blob signified that there was something in there that didn't traditionally go into ice cream. Check the ingredient list on a container of ice cream. You are likely to find some kind of food gum, perhaps several. It may even be listed as natural or organic. These are lovely words, conjuring a world-wise farmer in a straw hat, eschewing industrially produced fertilizers and genetically modified seedlings, somehow bringing forth natural locust bean gum and organic modified corn starch from the tilled earth. Or perhaps not. These descriptors are virtually meaningless. Far more important are the nouns that follow them.

Just because something is listed as natural or organic doesn't mean it belongs in your food. (Technically, you can also obtain natural or organic cocaine or arsenic, though I don't recommend it.) Food gums, like xanthan gum as it turns out, are almost always derived from natural substances. Modified food starches can be derived from organic, non-GMO plants. And lots of them are now included in your ice cream, even and especially nondairy ice cream that is marketed as somehow being better for you (it's not).

Though hard to find, there are ice creams without emulsifiers, most notably, Häagen-Dazs, which also happens to be delicious, if a little pricey (still, you have to read their ingredient labels, too, as not all flavors are free of emulsifiers). But price doesn't necessarily dictate quality in food these days. There are brands that are even more expensive than Häagen-Dazs, purporting to be somehow gourmet or artisan ice cream but chock-full of food gums and other ingredients found in the cheapest store brand. Like *natural* and *organic*, *gourmet* and *artisan* are marketing terms much more than they are signifiers of gut friendliness.

What about making your own? As a rainy-day activity, why not pick up some milk, cream, and sugar and get down to it? The stumbling block in what otherwise could be a fun project is the cream.

What's in Cream (Even "Organic" or "Natural" Cream)?

You may have a hard time finding unadulterated cream on store shelves (at least without a co-op market or dairy nearby) because without some kind of emulsifying agent, the pasteurization process causes the cream to separate as it sits in the store's refrigerator. So you either need fairly fresh pasteurized cream or really fresh unpasteurized cream to go additive-free. As a physician, I cannot recommend drinking unpasteurized cream. Pasteurization has prevented thousands of deaths and millions of illnesses. It isn't a bad thing. It just makes finding good cream a challenge. Listeria, the bacteria you can get from unpasteurized dairy, is worse than additives.

It's just too hard to be perfect, so we might as well start letting go here. Whole Foods has an in-house brand that is completely additive-free, but it doesn't seem to always be in stock. Like any pasteurized and additive-free heavy cream, it is prone to separate and can have chunks of milk fat solids that plop unpleasantly into your cup or dish when you pour it. Whipping the cream solves this problem, so I still buy it when it is available. Sometimes health food markets have a local creamery supply them with fresh cream that they do pasteurize. This is ideal. If you have this option, well, I'm jealous.

A good first step is to find creams without carrageenan. Some creams use only a small amount of one food gum (you can look down the list of ingredients for where the additive is positioned—farther down usually means less of it is used, at least in comparison to the other ingredients). A good second step is buying a cream with fewer gums. Horizon organic brand of heavy whipping cream (along with some other organic brands) has only gellan gum in it, as opposed to multiple other additives that many other brands include.

If we consider it possible that the quantity and mixture of substances consumed contribute to some of the trouble with ultra-processed foods (remember, it could be the dose that makes the poison), a dollop of heavy cream with only a little gum in it may be tolerable for most of us if we are unable to find a gum-free cream or if the slightly gloppy kind is unacceptable.

––––––––––

If you've given up dairy but haven't been diagnosed with an allergy to it or aren't fully lactose intolerant, you may want to give dairy another try—only this time without the additives. The same principle holds true for the next food category we are going to discuss—bread and grains.

Chapter 6

Bread and Grains

All sorrows are less with bread.

—*Miguel de Cervantes Saavedra*

Maryam, a forty-year-old woman whose family hails from Egypt, had been noting bowel troubles since her twenties, often suffering with cramping, bloating, and gas after a meal. Like many IBS patients, Maryam had cut out gluten from her diet about ten years earlier, finding some relief from her symptoms—though it was inconsistent. She was meticulous about avoiding gluten, but some days she felt like she had eaten it, although she was sure she hadn't, winding up with the same bowel troubles that had plagued her earlier. She began to restrict her diet more and more in search of relief. Then, she went to Egypt.

"I hadn't visited Egypt in years. And I thought, why is it that it seems like no one there has gluten problems? I thought, 'there is something different in the food in America that is causing problems.'"

Maryam decided to take a chance on the bread products in Egypt, and to her great surprise and delight her bowels were fine. Breads and other wheat-based items in Egypt didn't bother her one bit. She began to eat all foods without any restrictions and without incident. Upon returning to the US, Maryam decided to make her own bread from flour she had specially ordered—it promised to be minimally processed and pesticide-free. She, again, was fine. Given the high cost of that flour, I asked her to try homemade bread made with standard, all-purpose,

85

unbleached flour. She did and was happy to report back that, again, she was fine. She was also okay eating pasta and pastries, provided they didn't have additives in them. It turns out that gluten was never the problem for Maryam.

What If It Isn't Gluten After All?

Walking into the busy sandwich shop on Via de' Neri in Florence, I was immediately greeted by the warm, yeasty smell of freshly baked bread. After a minute or so of standing in the quickly moving line, an apron-clad, dark-haired man sped past holding a tray of still steaming giant ciabatta breads to ferry across the street to another shop. I turned to the right and from behind a glass plate I watched an identical ciabatta bread being piled high with fresh roast beef, cheese, and bright-red tomato slices that were about to be my lunch. When I brought the flour-dusted bread to my lips, I inhaled deeply, and crunched past the shell to the warm, soft interior.

I cannot think of a food I love more than freshly baked bread—the smell alone draws me into almost any shop or restaurant. Most cultures that have had historical access to wheat have their own fantastic takes on bread—Turkish, Indian, German, and, yes, Italian. It's hard to choose a favorite.

Unfortunately for about one in one hundred to two hundred Americans,[144] wheat-based bread is not an option. They have a condition called celiac disease. Celiac (for short) is not an allergy in the classic sense of the word—the cells responsible for allergic reactions aren't involved in this condition. Instead, celiac disease happens when the body mistakes the protein in wheat (also in barley and rye), known as gluten, for a foreign invader. The celiac sufferer's body then turns the attack on itself and destroys absorptive cells in the small intestine, making this an autoimmune disease. People with celiac need to avoid even the smallest amount of gluten to stay healthy. It is a serious problem. What we discuss next does not apply to anyone who has been diagnosed with celiac disease.

Gluten sensitivity is not the same as celiac disease. Unlike a patient with celiac, who will have characteristic flattening of the lining of their small intestines and antibodies detectible on a blood test, patients who have a suspected gluten sensitivity will have mostly normal-looking intestines and no such antibodies.

86

But they do feel better when avoiding gluten-containing foods.[145] Doctors don't fully understand this and have been looking for the cause of gluten sensitivity in these patients' immune systems. A study from the Mayo Clinic suggested that patients with certain immune system markers might be more susceptible to gluten sensitivity.[146] Others have proposed that gluten might not be the culprit in many or even most of these patients.

An Australian study put two groups of patients who thought they suffered from gluten sensitivity on a low-FODMAP diet and then gave them no-, low-, and high-gluten diets, finding no difference in bowel symptoms no matter the level of gluten consumed.[147] The authors proposed that perhaps substances other than the FODMAP groups of foods interact with gluten or that it might be something else entirely—perhaps fructans, which are also found in gluten-containing foods—that is the actual cause of symptoms.

Based on what I have seen in my practice and in myself, I tend to agree with the latter theory but have some doubt that fructans are to blame for all of us. Just as summertime or swimming was suspected to be a cause of polio before the virus that actually causes it was found (it just happened that the virus thrived during the summer and lived in kids' poop and we know what kids do in pools), gluten and fructans could quite possibly be co-travelers in the bread we eat. Because celiac disease is such a serious condition and one in which gluten is clearly the culprit, it initially made sense to look to gluten as the cause of milder gastrointestinal symptoms in people without celiac. But there have been too many dead ends to continue along this path for many patients.

Now, let me be clear. Some people have found that they feel undeniably better when avoiding gluten. I am not telling them to stop doing this. However, if you are like many who sometimes feel better and then sometimes don't when avoiding gluten, if you occasionally feel worse and just aren't sure, it may be worth a try to see if it might not be gluten after all.

I happily consumed gluten-rich, crusty breads with pillowy interiors in Italy, and was absolutely fine. They certainly had fructans in them too, since fructans occur naturally in wheat. But like Maryam, who was fine in Egypt, I suffered when I resumed eating bread after I came back to the US. The gluten was the same or at least pretty similar in both countries. The fructans were the same. But there were other ingredients that were quite different.

We have pretty much transformed bread, which is a global food staple, traditionally made with water, wheat, and some kind of rising agent, into a soft substance resembling bread. But bread is also made with a host of other non-bread ingredients. The ingredients to which I am referring have no nutritious value but increase the shelf life of the loaf—sometimes by weeks at a time. This is good for bread makers, supermarkets, and, quite frankly, our pocketbooks (the longer something lasts, the cheaper it is), but it can be bad for our intestines and perhaps the rest of our bodies.

The Real Trouble with Commercial Breads and Pastas

Many patients with bowel distress quickly observe that eating commercially made bread does not agree with them. But when encouraged to try homemade loaves or sometimes sourdough (which usually has fewer to no additives), the problems with gluten can disappear. Is this because there is somehow less gluten in sourdough breads? Or possibly fewer fructans? Maybe, but this has never really been adequately demonstrated, and the type of flour used—bread flour versus all-purpose versus wheat—may have a greater impact on how much gluten is actually in the bread. This still leaves the puzzle of why a homemade loaf using off-the-shelf flour and yeast (or the loaves I had in Italy) doesn't bother some people who previously thought they were sensitive to gluten. In medicine, we often quote the nineteenth-century physician William Osler, who said, "listen to your patient, he's telling you the diagnosis."[148] People are telling us there is something not right with commercially made bread. We would be wise to listen.

So if it's not the gluten (at least not for everyone), what could it be? A loaf of supermarket bread certainly has quite a few non-bread ingredients to consider. A quick scan of the back of a bag of commercially made bread is likely to reveal mono- and diglycerides. As previously mentioned, these are emulsifying agents, and they are in countless numbers of ultra-processed foods these days. Mono- and diglycerides may not be the worst of the additive microbiome disrupters,[149] but they are best avoided because they often make an appearance in ultra-processed baked goods that seem to impact patients with IBS and those with metabolic and blood sugar issues.

So what bread can we eat? The simple answer is the freshly baked kind from a real bakery or your own kitchen. Okay, stop laughing. I'm not suggesting you become an amateur bread baker. I've tried. It takes a while, and by *a while* I mean an entire afternoon or even longer. For the weekend hobbyists for whom baking is a treat, learn to bake your own real bread. It's truly the best solution. Alternatively, if you have an independently owned scratch bakery in your neighborhood, consider yourself lucky and support it if you are financially able to do so.

If there isn't such a shop nearby, getting unadulterated bread can prove to be a difficult task. Some co-op markets and farmers markets carry delicious loaves, but these can be pricey, sometimes available only during limited hours, and unpredictable in their supply.

Of all the shopping and cooking modifications I've had to make, bread has presented the greatest challenge. I'll occasionally spring for a sourdough loaf at a natural food market. Though please be aware that natural food marts often have more adulterated breads than unadulterated ones, so read labels there, too, perhaps even more closely because you may not be expecting additives to be included in the products from an expensive market supposedly selling fresher and healthier items.

The ingredient list for most breads should only include wheat, water, yeast (if not a sourdough where it may be called a starter), salt, eggs (if an egg bread like challah), and butter (if a brioche or croissant-like bread). Label reading gets much quicker after a few weeks of finding your new favorites. And remember these loaves don't have the additives in them to keep them fresh for weeks, so you will have to eat them quickly (not generally a problem with good bread) or freeze them to eat later.

While you are being careful with bread, also be careful with bread crumbs. Texture is a big deal in food and a quick way to get added texture is to bread things. Bread crumbs are great for coating chicken, fish, and sometimes even veggies like eggplant and zucchini, which kids might not otherwise eat. They also help hold meatballs and meat loaves together. But, disappointingly, bread crumbs can also contain mono- and diglycerides as well as several other additives. The lack of additives in several brands of bread crumbs makes one feel as though the choice to add them is somewhat arbitrary. The product still works great without additives. And since there are plenty of brands that don't include these unnecessary ingredients, a little label reading will go a long way here. Many products seem to be priced the same and work identically in dishes, their only difference being the addition of potentially gut-roiling additives.

While bread is the biggest offender, those with presumed gluten sensitivities will say that it is not only bread but other gluten-containing items that they struggle with—wraps, pastas, cakes, cookies, all of them tarred with the same brush. Again, gluten is a likely co-traveler in these items, not necessarily the actual perpetrator of the GI distress for some of us. Any food that stays soft for a prolonged period of time probably stays that way due to one, or possibly more, microbiome-disrupting additive. A good rule to follow is, if it's soft and shelf-stable, check that label!

Conversely, foods that are sold in hard, dried, or crunchy form are often okay, precisely because they contain none of the additives that are needed to keep them soft on the refrigerator shelf. (Of course, that's not a blanket statement.) When it comes to pasta, the dried, boxed ones are almost universally fine, made with just flour and water and sometimes egg. The soft ones on the shelf or in the refrigerated aisles, though? Probably not okay. Frozen pastas? Sometimes okay. Read those labels carefully or just save your money and stick with the good, cheap, old-fashioned dried stuff. If you are going gluten-free, be careful of alternative grain pastas as these often need binders to keep them together. Although alternative grain products try to market themselves as healthier, they rarely are.

If you were troubled by pasta in the past, possibly consider that the culprit might have been whatever the pasta was covered in, not the pasta itself, and baby-step your way back. Start with a simple dried pasta and just coat it in a little olive oil or butter. If that doesn't bother you and you are a tomato sauce fan, try that next time—most jarred tomato sauces are just fine (but check the label just to be safe). Then throw some Parmesan you've grated yourself (this is really important) on top. This is basically the pasta dish I had in Italy at the Autogrill, and it helped me re-embrace many foods I thought I'd have to give up forever.

When I realized that my trouble wasn't with gluten so I didn't have to give up any specific food, only specific additives, I decided to begin at the beginning. Literally, the beginning of the day, since breakfast is—at least for us in the United States—often a carbohydrate-heavy affair.

It's a Wrap, but What's in It?

If foods that are soft and shelf-stable are problematic, wraps and soft tortillas are trouble and then some. Marketed as low-carb alternatives to bread, they are that, but they are also full of the monoglycerides, lecithins, and other dough conditioners that have infiltrated our bread supply. Because they need to stay soft, it's also fairly common to see food gums used in tortillas as well. Luckily, you can sometimes find frozen flour or alternative grain tortillas in the freezer aisle without additives. They stay fresh because they are frozen.

If in doubt, stick to crunchy, corn-based shells—these should only have a few basic ingredients: corn, lime, oil, and salt. Hard and crunchy food products generally need little but salt and an airtight environment to keep them shelf-stable, but there are no guarantees of unadulterated food here, either. Do not be misled by the front of the package that may declare the product to be preservative-free or all-natural.

Breakfast Cereal: Big Trouble in Little Boxes

The stereotypical American breakfast dates back to the late 1800s with Dr. John Harvey Kellogg's introduction of corn flakes.[150] Before Kellogg's invention, breakfast consisted of the previous night's leftovers or perhaps a piece of bread and cheese. Often, there was meat involved. Dr. Kellogg, however, was a devout Seventh-day Adventist and avowed vegetarian. A medical doctor who obtained his degree from the University of Michigan, he was also a proponent of the clean-living movement, whose tenets might sound familiar to clean-living folks today—no alcohol, caffeine, or tobacco.[151] Another stated goal of the cereal maker was to curb sexual appetites (this makes sense when we consider how unsexy corn flakes are). In short, John Harvey Kellogg was probably not a lot of fun at parties. It should probably also be mentioned that he was a noted eugenicist and racist, so we should take his recommendations with a grain of salt. Even so, a few of his nutrition ideas didn't completely miss the mark.

Kellogg was a proponent of whole grains and eschewed sweet foods. The original corn flakes probably tasted more like the box it now comes in rather than the sugar-sweetened stuff we recognize today. But Kellogg's brother, who maybe was more fun at parties, soon took over and figured out that sugar sells, and the other, quickly multiplying cereal manufacturers soon followed his lead.[152]

After the highly successful introduction of sugar, and later high-fructose corn syrup, the cereal additives just kept coming. With an emphasis on marketing and convenience, more traditional breakfast foods didn't stand a chance. And so today we have an entire aisle in the grocery store devoted to ultra-processed breakfast bits delivered in brightly colored cardboard boxes.

Unfortunately, besides truckloads of sweetness delivered in the form of high-fructose corn syrup, many contain a potentially worse insult to GI health—maltodextrin. Maltodextrin is another altered sugar compound, which is used as a stabilizing and bulking agent. Besides cereal, maltodextrin is added to a lot of foods to enhance their flavor and shelf life. On the face of it, it sounds like a great idea to help reduce the amount of sugar added and to keep food around longer, therefore making it cheaper. Sadly, as with anything in life, if something sounds too good to be true, it probably is. It turns out that maltodextrin can cause spikes in blood sugar, may promote growth of less than favorable bad gut bacteria, and contribute to gut inflammation.[153] Researchers have shown that maltodextrin facilitates the adherence of potentially invasive *E. coli* to the small intestinal cells.[154] The 2021 guidelines issued by the IOIBD advise patients with Crohn's disease and those with UC to avoid maltodextrin.

Something about the intestinal cells of patients with Crohn's disease may cause bacteria to attach more securely when they are able to proliferate in a maltodextrin-rich environment. Maltodextrin also may be problematic in people who don't have this potential genetic predisposition in their cells, since it has been implicated as a promoter of the metabolic syndrome and as a potential trigger for IBS.[155]

But you will have to pry the cereal box out of my cold, sleepy hands. One kid won't get out of bed. The other can't find her shoes. And we all need to get going! Mornings are challenging in most homes, and cereal provides a cheap and quick solution—one that most kids over the age of six can handle getting for themselves. So go ahead and eat that bowl of cereal, but be careful which cereals you stock your pantry shelves with. As Dr. Monteiro has suggested, try to replace the ultra-processed food with something less processed. Simple breakfast cereals without gut-disturbing additives can be found on any supermarket shelf. Brands like Barbara's or Kashi promote their products as simpler and less processed. To be safe, even though I've been impressed by these companies, read their labels, too—companies change hands and formulas can be altered. As an added bonus, a lot of these cereals (though not all) have less added sugar—something we all should probably cut back on where possible. You can throw a sliced banana or some berries into your bowl if you need more of a sweet taste in the morning, plus you'll be getting some more whole, nutritious food into your diet—not a bad idea for all of us.

If you want to go even more whole food–based, there is always oatmeal (with some caveats—you aren't surprised, are you?). Oatmeal is supposed to be simple and healthy. It's the perfect food for people short on time (read: pretty much all of us). Oatmeal is great! How could we mess up oatmeal? It's oats. And water. And maybe a little sugar or cinnamon or raisins. And yet, we have. In addition to the ingredients you might expect, individually packaged oatmeal (and by extension, oatmeal at quick-serve restaurants, or any restaurant for that matter) can contain emulsifiers or thickening agents in the form of modified food starches and food gums.

I began to wonder why these additives had made it into oatmeal packets in the first place. Oatmeal thickens up when you cook it in water, making its own natural carbohydrate-based gel by breaking down its naturally occurring starch as it heats up. The hotter the oatmeal gets, the thicker it gets (up to a point).[156] If this is already a naturally occurring phenomenon, why add anything to it?

The answer here is basically the answer to most of the ultra-processed food mysteries. The additive either makes the product cheaper to produce or saves the consumer time. In this case, adding a thickening agent reduces the amount of time needed to cook the oatmeal to attain the most desirable consistency. Grab a packet of oatmeal with the additives, add water, microwave for a minute, and voilà—breakfast! Sounds great except for the problems the additives may cause.

So do we really need additives? Well, without additives it would take more time to cook the oatmeal—another minute or two or three perhaps to achieve the desired consistency. And then you'd have to add your own sweeteners or fruit if you like that sort of thing. A bowl of oatmeal is now a five-minute chore instead of a one-minute task. It doesn't sound like a lot, but mornings can be harried, especially with kids.

What if you could cut that down to two or three minutes? And what if you could also get a stomachache-free morning as part of the bargain? That should easily be worth an extra minute or two. So buy plain oats, avoiding the little individual packages that often have the thickening and emulsifying agents in them. As a bonus, you will save a little money. If you miss the convenience of premade oatmeal packets, here are a couple of ways to DIY:

- Prepare small baggies or containers in advance for the week. Put ½ cup of oats into each container. Add some dried fruit, a sprinkle of sugar, cinnamon, or whatever you like. When you want oatmeal, pour the contents into a bowl, add 1 cup of water, and microwave it just like you did the little packets, perhaps for a minute or so longer to achieve the desired consistency.

- Try overnight oats. You can prepare them the night before (you can even make a larger batch and enjoy it for a few days). There are many recipes to be found online for overnight oats, but the basic idea is to take oats and soak them in milk or yogurt (either dairy or a nondairy alternative) without additives in a jar overnight in the fridge. Generally, a 1-to-1 ratio of oats to liquid works. People add nuts or fruit or warm it up in the morning to get more creative. Oatmeal is like that sturdy shelf in your house that you keep piling stuff onto—it can support almost anything.

Pancakes and Waffles

Some people just don't like oatmeal, and that's okay. Frozen breakfast staples can offer a kid-friendly breakfast for busy families. It turns out that frozen waffles and pancakes are pretty similar, with the more expensive organic or whole grain options having many of the same additives as the mainstream and more affordable ones, sometimes even more! Mainstream waffles and pancakes often have high-fructose corn syrup, which in small quantities may be okay, and soy lecithin, which may also be okay in small quantities. However, if you are really trying to figure out what is upsetting your system or trying to avoid ultra-processed additives, you might want to skip these to start out.

If you (or your kids) simply must have a hot pancake breakfast to face the day, consider making pancakes from scratch on the weekend and freezing a few extra for the rest of the week. Pancakes are not at all hard to make from scratch—flour, eggs, milk, a little sugar, salt, oil, and baking powder. There's an easy recipe at the end of this book. Mixes really save only seconds, are pricey, and have succeeded solely based on heavy marketing. They also contain emulsifiers and dough conditioners that you absolutely don't need. You can make better pancakes yourself without the gut-roiling additives. Store the extras in a freezer bag after they have completely cooled, then defrost them for a few seconds in the microwave on a busy morning.

Just like dairy, gluten may not be the villain it's been made out to be for many of us. Carbohydrates, on the other hand, are a little more complicated. If you are struggling with diabetes or metabolic syndrome, your body may be having a hard time dealing with carbs, especially the processed kind.

When I say *eat everything*, I mean it. But that doesn't mean eat everything with abandon. If you've been told to watch your blood sugar, that includes carbohydrates, which is what grains mostly are. The good news is that the less processed the carbohydrate is, the more slowly your blood sugar will rise when you consume it (more on this in the next chapter). Not all carbohydrates are created equal. It turns out that the carbohydrates and other components found in most fruits and vegetables are nourishing for us and our microbiomes. So why are some of them getting a bad rap?

Chapter 7

Fruits and Vegetables

Live each season as it passes; breathe the air,
drink the drink, taste the fruit...

—*Henry David Thoreau*

Isaac is a thirty-five-year-old man who felt pretty good most of the time and didn't have any medical diagnoses. He was in the office for a routine checkup and was wondering what he could do to stay well. The advice he had been getting from friends and the internet was often conflicting and overly burdensome. I asked him what he had heard. He took a deep breath and began.

"I know saturated fat is bad, but what if it comes from coconuts or cashews? Plants are good, right?"

He didn't pause for me to respond.

"Eggs were bad, but then they were good, and now they are just okay, and I shouldn't have more than two a week? But maybe all animal protein is bad, and I should just be vegan, but I don't like beans or lentils, and, quite frankly, I don't want to be vegan." He stopped and shrugged. "Why do the experts keep changing their minds so much and also, what are the superfoods I should be eating?"

Isaac was a successful engineer and led an extremely organized life. He belonged to a gym and exercised three to four times a week. He had a drink or two on the weekends and had never smoked anything. He had already ascertained that he should definitely be eating more vegetables. But even the advice he was getting about vegetables seemed confusing. How much was enough, and could it be that some vegetables were actually bad for you, as he had also heard? That the experts kept changing their minds and offered conflicting advice bothered him on both a personal and a professional level. His job depended on him being precise and getting it right the first time. Why couldn't the food scientists get it together?

The problem, as I explained to him, is that we have spent the last one hundred years focused on the components of food and not on the actual foods in their entirety. This is called nutritional reductionism, and when we didn't even know what food was made up of, it made some sense. Once we were able to identify individual dietary components like carbohydrates, fats, protein, vitamins, minerals, fiber, and cholesterol, we started basing advice and guidelines on those. That wasn't wrong. We need a certain amount of vitamins, minerals, and all the rest for our bodies to function properly. The knowledge that was gained by nutritional reductionism was necessary, but we are learning that it isn't sufficient information on which to build a truly healthy diet.

However, the food industry built their businesses by focusing the foods they were making on meeting those requirements—stuffing their new ultra-processed products with vitamins and fiber and then calling them healthy. The problem is that people don't eat vitamins and fiber in isolation. We eat food, and the way actual food behaves in our bodies is not the same as when the distilled components were studied. So we have wound up with a diet composed of an overgrowth of additives and a paucity of the whole foods that actually protect our bodies from disease. Focusing on just the components of what we are eating in isolation has thus led to confusion and jaw-dropping rates of noncommunicable diseases in areas of the world that have embraced nutritional reductionism.[157]

It's not wrong to ask which vitamins we should be getting more of or how much of a dietary component might be too much, but before searching for superfoods or delving into the polyphenol amounts in one berry versus another, we need to take a broader view. Sure, some fruits, vegetables, grains, and nuts may be better than others, but for most of us, simply trying to get rid of ultra-processed foods and eating a whole-food diet (as much as possible) should be the foundation. There is a deluge of information out there on which superfoods to trim your diet with, but that won't make a huge difference if there's not a strong base to begin with. To do that, we have to move away from nutritional reductionism and look at whole foods.

Looking at the Whole Food

As previously mentioned, substances that occur naturally in whole fruits and vegetables may act differently than those that are added to foods during ultra-processing. To see why, let's consider something called the glycemic index.

Glycemic index is roughly a measure of how quickly a food item drives up blood sugar relative to a gram of glucose, which was given the value of 100. The lower the number, the slower food is digested, and the slower blood sugar rises. The higher the number, the faster food is digested, and the faster blood sugar rises. An orange has a glycemic index of 43. Orange juice has a glycemic index of 50. A whole orange has naturally occurring fiber that is removed when just the juice is consumed. To make things a little more complicated, take a potato. A plain boiled potato has a glycemic index of 78. But process the potato into a powder to create an instant mashed potato ultra-processed food, and the glycemic index shoots up to 87.[158]

Whole foods generally are digested more slowly, and this can have a major impact on blood sugar control—it's why my patients with diabetes who counted carbohydrates did so much better when they cut out ultra-processed foods in favor of whole foods. Counting carbs wasn't enough—that's nutritionally reductive. Looking at the whole foods turned out to be equally important.

The speed at which we digest food doesn't just impact blood sugar—it affects our entire GI tract. It turns out that when you eat an apple, the fiber is still stuck in the cell walls of the fruit as it passes through your small intestine and arrives in your large intestine. The cell wall needs to be broken down before the organisms in our gut can make use of the fiber-fuel, so the bacteria in the large intestine have some more work to do to break it down. There may also be a variety of additional components in the whole food that affect digestion in other ways that scientists are still working out. In a study comparing prunes to a fiber supplement called psyllium, prunes actually helped people with constipation more than the psyllium even though there was an equivalent amount of fiber in both the prunes and the supplement. So there was something else in the whole food, or something in the way the fiber was incorporated into the actual food, that made it work better than the supplement.[159]

The Fiber Fiasco

If we can't eat enough naturally occurring fiber in the form of fruits and veggies, the thinking goes, at least we have food gums, which, due to their chemical structure and inability to be digested (by us, not by our microbiomes) are classified as a type of fiber. If you are eating an ultra-processed food labeled "High in Fiber," it may have a type of food gum added to it. (Remember chicory root fiber, aka inulin, which we discussed in chapter 3? That's a common food gum.) Our understanding of the way our guts and our microbiomes process different fibers is poor at best and probably wrong at worst. Simply put, all fiber is not created equal. And different fibers' effects on your body are not the same. In some cases, additives that have been dumped into the fiber category are probably not acting quite like the natural fibers encased in their plant homes and may be doing some harm.

When fiber is added to packaged foods in the form of food gums or cellulose or whatever new and exciting fiber is being added this week, it has no cell wall and digestion can happen earlier in the gastrointestinal tract and more rapidly.[160] This not only changes how the food is absorbed into our bodies (affecting the rate of rise of blood sugar demonstrated by the glycemic index), but where and how fast food is broken down probably has an effect on how quickly and which bacteria grows in our guts.[161]

Traditionally, when more of the plant cell wall needed to be broken down, bacteria wouldn't have access to much of the food until it arrived in the large intestine. Now, more food is ready to be consumed by the microbiome in the small intestine. Although we have been removing plant cell walls for hundreds of years—for instance, milling whole grains into powdery white flour—the rate at which we are now providing our gut residents with more easily accessible fiber-food that can be digested earlier is increasing exponentially. This may allow for territory expansion of not-so-friendly gut bacteria, according to some researchers—very different from the promotion of beneficial bacteria in the colon by eating the fiber encased in whole foods.[162] So eating whole fruits and vegetables provides nutrition not only for us, but also for our microbial gut inhabitants and in the place they are supposed to be consuming them.

It's easy enough to tell someone to eat more fruits and vegetables. A parent or grandparent probably told you to do that. But what if it is a struggle? Some vegetables and fruits just don't seem to agree with all of us. If you haven't been told to specifically avoid a particular item, consider that—like the example of pasta in the previous chapter—it may not be the fruit or veggie, but what we are putting on it that is causing the trouble.

Salad Problems Solved

I didn't see much in the way of salad dressing in Italy. Greens would sometimes, but not always, be served with small bottles of good olive oil and balsamic vinegar. The vegetables were bright and fresh: tomatoes were ripe and sweet, dripping with their own juices; lettuces were crisp and flavorful and sometimes peppery. I quickly surmised that the reason there were no dressings in Italy was because there was no need for them—the salad already had all the flavors it needed.

Italy has a great deal of volcanic soil, rich in minerals and able to hold water well, in which to grow its produce, so that certainly helps. But probably a bigger contributor to the glory of those Italian fruits and vegetables is that they are grown nearby, so they can be picked at the height of ripeness and enjoyed soon thereafter. The restaurants we visited in Italy offered only what was being harvested that week. Period. Do not ask for broccoli when it isn't in season. And be prepared to eat a lot of artichokes when they are coming in by the bushel.

April in Rome features the old Jewish quarter sidewalks lined with men deftly wielding small knives, peeling artichokes, trying to entice customers into the establishments behind them to partake of the fried goodness. *You see?* their fast-moving hands are imploring wordlessly. *The freshness of our artichokes will not be beat.* Although you previously had no intention of doing so, you go inside the restaurant and order artichokes. They are some of the best artichokes you have ever eaten in your life—even without dressing or sauce.

In the US, we are incredibly fortunate. Produce is trucked or flown in from all over the world and delivered to our supermarkets. A variety of fruits and vegetables are available year-round. Want watermelon in January? You will probably be able to find it. An apple in the sweltering heat of summer? No problem. Your favorite salad at your trusty chain restaurant need never have its ingredients change. The salad will look roughly like the picture on the menu wherever and whenever you go. Convenience and predictability are useful in a country as big as the United States. I like the comfort of being in an unfamiliar city and being able to pop into a restaurant where I already know the menu. I know how much it will cost and just what the food will taste like.

But reliability comes with additional, unexpected costs. The human and environmental costs are beyond the scope of this book but must at least be acknowledged: mass-producing fruits and vegetables out of season in the US involves terrible working conditions for mostly undocumented harvesters, and requires tremendous amounts of herbicides and pesticides. The cost that is relevant to our discussion, though, is the one we wind up paying for in flavor (and possibly in nutrition—see the box on page 107).

Fruits and vegetables often have to be harvested before they have fully ripened in order to be shipped. That means they will have fewer natural sugars, though they may look ripe due to forced ripening. They won't taste the same as a freshly picked produce because most of their natural sugars are still in the form of starch.[163]

My Soviet-born father unknowingly, but brilliantly, summed up the phenomenon by declaring that a tomato (or other untimely picked fruit or vegetable) tastes like a potato because, well, a potato is made up of mostly bland, long-chain starches, and so are unripe fruits and vegetables.

The solution to this flavorless dilemma is simple: add sauce. Or dressing. Add anything to brighten the taste of our potato-like produce. And so, our salads are smothered. Because avoiding dressing has been a big help to my GI system, I now ask for salads in restaurants without dressing. The servers almost always still bring it on the side. One went so far as to ask, "Have you ever had our salad without dressing? You probably won't like it."

Truth be told, I'm not crazy about most salads in the US without dressing. But I dislike what makes its way into most bottled or preprepared dressings even more. Almost every prepackaged dressing I can think of is an emulsion—a

Vegetable-Based Dips and Spreads

Besides being put off by foods with ingredients that separate, it turns out that truly natural foods can be somewhat unpredictable and trickier to work with. So even some high-priced brands resort to emulsifiers and stabilizers to keep their products looking fresh.

Natural acids are a great way of preserving some dips and spreads without additional additives. Most commercially available salsas are full of natural acid and stay fresh on the supermarket shelf for a long time. The same can be true for guacamole.

Price doesn't always indicate quality in our food anymore, and it's best not to assume that you are avoiding emulsifiers and other additives by buying seemingly healthy plant-based sides and dips. A chef-branded product might contain modified food starch, whereas a cheaper version may have none. The ubiquitous brand of hummus available in all my area supermarkets is just chickpeas, tahini, and lemon, whereas the gourmet brand is filled with food gums.

As with other foods, if you aren't making it yourself, check the label and ignore words like *gourmet* or *chef made* just like you should be ignoring *natural* and *organic*. The words and the price aren't a guarantee of anything, even—and maybe especially—when eating plant-based foods.

mixture of fat-soluble and water-soluble ingredients. If the dressing isn't consumed relatively quickly, it will begin to separate. While that's not a huge problem—you can just shake or stir the liquid to get the ingredients to mix again—it can be unsightly, especially if the dressing is meant to sit for months on a shelf. So additives are put into most dressings to avoid this phenomenon. Let an oil-based dressing sit for a few minutes. If it doesn't start to separate, be suspicious.

The main gut-riling culprits in dressings are food gums, as in ice creams, and modified food starches, as in some bread products. Even organic or natural dressings probably have xanthan gum or another food gum in them. Does that mean we have to eat bland, dry salads? No. It means we have to get creative.

Happily, in this case, it's easy! Because unlike bread or ice cream, which may require some time to create from scratch, dressings are incredibly simple to make at home. By having garlic (and a garlic press), citrus in the form of lemons and limes, Dijon mustard, olive oil, vinegars, and a few dried herbs and spices on hand, you pretty much eliminate the need for bottled marinades and dressings. I'm not sure when this bit of culinary information was lost, but this is knowledge worth reclaiming. All of these ingredients naturally keep for a long time (even citrus, properly stored, will last a few weeks), are cheap (unless you spring for the pricey mustard), and can be turned into amazing flavorful dressings in minutes (and then stored for several days in the fridge). Here are some ideas:

- Try the good old combo of oil and vinegar.
- Mix equal parts balsamic vinegar and Dijon mustard for a creamy dressing with a kick—it takes less than a minute to do this.
- For an easy Caesar-like dressing (hold the anchovy), get a mayonnaise without additives (found in almost any supermarket and should have only oil, eggs, mustard, lemon juice, vinegar, and some spices in the ingredient list), then add some lemon juice, crushed garlic, Dijon mustard, and a hearty pinch of black pepper.
- For a Greek-style dressing, combine olive oil, lemon juice, crushed or minced garlic, and oregano.

Because these dressings have fresh garlic in them, they will only last up to five days. If you want them to last longer, you can use garlic powder instead (just substitute ⅛ teaspoon of garlic powder for each garlic clove). Doing this will help your vinaigrette last up to two weeks in the fridge—remember that homemade dressings must be stored in the refrigerator. See Appendix C for more specific ideas for dressings.

You can take your quest for delicious veggies a step further than DIY dressings. We grow food in the US. If you have the means, buying local seasonal vegetables and fruits isn't terribly difficult if you have access to farmers' markets or even farm delivery/pick-up services, also called Community Supported Agriculture. Sometimes it's actually cheaper since you aren't also paying high transportation costs for your food to be flown in from across the globe.

Fruit Is Your Friend (Usually)

Fruit is good for you. Really good for you. This is another place where the low-FODMAP concept falls flat. It cuts out many healthy fruits and veggies and starves the microbiome of the important fiber prebiotics in whole fruits. Eating whole fruits and veggies has myriad health benefits, especially for the gastrointestinal system. Avoiding them is not sound advice for most people.

You may notice that fruits and vegetables that have caused problems in the past don't anymore when you cut out emulsifiers and thickeners. It's possible you could notice a difference within days. Your microbiome is constantly turning over. Thousands of your gut bacteria just reproduced in the time it took you to read this sentence. So you can start to eat everything relatively quickly once you eliminate the additives. In one study, it took a total of one day for subjects' microbiomes to change dramatically when a new diet was introduced.[164] This explains why after only a day of eating in Italy, I felt like I had a brand-new gut. It was basically because I did. Two days off the healthier diet in that study saw

Eat Everything Easy Meal Idea: Salad in a Jar

Eat more veggies is solid advice for many of us and having things ready to go helps. Salads can be prepared in advance, and several can be made at a time. Cut up a head or two of lettuce, some tomatoes, cucumbers, peppers, or whatever veggies you enjoy and have on hand. Throw them into three or four airtight containers. Hardboil and peel a few eggs, and toss them into a baggie. Drain and rinse some canned chickpeas to have in another container. These items tossed in at the last minute along with a slice or two of cheese (check that it's just milk, salt, and enzymes) or maybe a handful of chicken from last night's dinner, and you have lunch! This might also be a good time to use up some of your deli meat or tuna salad, too. The only thing left to do is to dress your salad (this should definitely be done at the last possible moment so the lettuce doesn't get soggy and limp).

participants' microbiomes reverting back to their original composition. This also explains why I felt miserable again shortly after returning to the US and reverted back to my additive-laden diet.

Which fruits are best? Well, I could argue about sugar content and glycemic index and fiber content and all sorts of nutritionally reductive things . . . but I said I wasn't going to do that. As far as I'm concerned, if the fruit comes to you intact, looking the same way it did when it was picked, although maybe with a little less dirt, it's great. (That is, unless you are struggling with your blood sugar, in which case I encourage you to discuss with your doctor or dietician how much fruit you should be eating. Likewise, if you are struggling with an active bout of colitis, you need to do what your gastroenterologist and dietician advise with regard to fiber-rich foods.)

What about fruit juice? As an occasional treat, it's fine. Remember that juice is a big fructose load without the fiber that a whole fruit provides, so it's not the same for your blood sugar and should be avoided if you struggle with that. A large quantity of juice can be tough for the gut to handle as well. Besides the naturally occurring fructose, additives are frequently put into juice and are not always listed on the label. When you see "100 Percent Juice" on the label, most often food manufacturers have added additional flavor enhancers to the juice. Though lawsuits have been brought against manufacturers to try to force them to list everything that goes into a bottle of juice, they've mostly failed.[165] So add misleading labeling to a host of other reasons to avoid juice.

Can you squeeze the juice yourself? Absolutely! You can still have juice and by forcing yourself to work for it, you'll wind up seeing it as a special treat, which it really should be.

Better than juicing is throwing whole fruit into a blender and making it into a smoothie. Note that most smoothie places don't actually do this. Instead they substitute the more expensive and prone-to-spoilage fresh fruit juices with other ingredients you may be trying to avoid. If you can't verify all the ingredients in your smoothie (beware of anything called a blend), make your own.

Making your own smoothies can be a lot cheaper than buying them. Basic blenders can be as inexpensive as $20 or $30, and more expensive options can be considered an excellent investment for making all kinds of homemade (and additive-free) foods. Smoothies are a great breakfast addition or afternoon snack and can even be full meals if made heartier with protein additions such as nut butter, chia seeds, or yogurt.

While breakfast is a great time to incorporate fruit into a diet, people attempting weight loss may want to make sure to add some protein, too (again, there are lots of books on this so I won't spend too much time here, but I'll simplify and say that having some protein in a meal will probably keep you full longer). Eating fruit combined with a source of protein is a great way to start the day.

What About Frozen, Dried, or Canned Produce?

We often think fresh is best, and it probably is. But truly fresh fruits and vegetables would have to come from your own garden or a nearby farm. After produce is harvested, it slowly becomes depleted of some of its nutrients. Frozen fruits and vegetables are usually picked at their peak, and the freezing process may help preserve some of their nutrients.[166] Canning, as long as a whole bunch of sugar or salt or other preservatives aren't added, does much the same. In fact, a 2015 study suggested that eaters of nutrient-dense canned foods (like fruits and vegetables) have improved nutrient intake over people who eat fewer canned foods.[167] And as long as you watch the preservatives in dried fruits, those can be a great source of nutrition as well. The main idea is to eat lots of produce in any form it's tastiest and easiest for you to do so. Remember not to get too caught up in the minutia and lose sight of the big picture: unprocessed or minimally processed plants are good for you.

A Word About Food Intolerance Testing

Finally, please beware of direct-to-consumer tests that purport to be able to tell you which foods you are intolerant of, either by examining a sample of blood or hair or something else. These tests are becoming increasingly popular and suggest that by cutting out healthy real foods, especially specific plants, from your diet, you will feel better. An NBC news senior correspondent took several of these tests and found that the results didn't correlate much with one another.[168] This isn't to say that intolerances and allergies to plants aren't real, only that if you think you have an intolerance or allergy, please see a board-certified allergist or gastroenterologist. And if you don't, try to embrace fruits and vegetables—they will love you and your microbiome right back.

Chapter 8

Meat, Poultry, Eggs, and Other Proteins

When people you greatly admire appear to be thinking deep thoughts, they probably are thinking about lunch.

—Douglas Adams

Plant-based diets have been gaining in popularity. According to the *New York Times*, while only 6 percent of Americans in 2019 identified as vegetarians, nearly 40 percent were trying to eat more plant-based foods.[169] That means they still may include some meat or other animal products in their diets. It also means that more than 60 percent of Americans are not trying to eat a plant-based diet.

Many excellent arguments make a great case for eating more plant-based foods. And in my family, we are trying. And by *we*, I mean me. My husband still fancies himself a pitmaster. It's where he finds joy. Plants are important, but so is joy and so is honoring tradition.

In my childhood neighborhood in Miami, my Argentinian American neighbor built his own brick barbeque. As special as it was, I merely recognized it as part of my neighbor's backyard. Meat was often cooked on it, and as luck would have it I was best friends with his daughter, so I got to partake in the feasts, too. My introduction to Cuban American food culture was a metal box called a *caja china*, which is used to roast an entire pig for celebrations. A cookout is a Southern and African American cultural touchstone. All this to say, eating animal products makes up an important part of a lot of traditional diets. But they were unlikely to have been eaten in large quantities, regularly, or by most people, so we probably shouldn't gorge ourselves on them, either.

Most of us can eat animal products in moderation and as careful label readers.* The prepared and packaged stuff can contain premade marinades with a lot of the additives we are trying to avoid. This chapter is all about how to eat proteins—and I'll start with a special note for those of us who are eating plant-based foods in case you want to skip right to dessert in chapter 9.

Vegetarian Proteins

My grandmother was a vegetarian. Though she never spoke about it, it was known family lore that after she had survived World War II, she never wanted to be responsible for the death of a living creature. Thus, she was vegetarian as long as I had known her and long before the food supply was infiltrated with an enormous amount of additives.

People adhering to vegetarian or even vegan diets isn't new. Long-established religions like Hinduism and Jainism encourage their followers to avoid eating animals. So what if you don't want to actually eat everything? Well, like people for thousands of years, you don't have to. But you do have to be particularly careful and perhaps slightly more adventurous about your eating.

Alternative meat and milk products are likely to be ultra-processed and full of the additives that I have been encouraging you to avoid, but not all of them are. For example, all veggie burgers are not created equal. They can be highly processed or made of minimally processed beans and grains. The same goes for soy-based proteins. Tofu and tempeh contain few ingredients, while soy protein fake meats tend to contain the additives we should be avoiding. Eating a plant-based diet is great. Eating more ultra-processed stuff isn't.

---

* Since I've commented on the ethical difficulties with the way we harvest produce in the US, I'd be remiss if I didn't also comment on the issues around animal farming for food, which are myriad. Factory farming has been noted to contribute to climate change, deforestation, antibiotic resistance, cruelty to the animals, loss of family farming and its resultant impact on rural communities. We can make choices to help minimize these impacts if we are meat eaters. Many resources are available to investigate this further if it is a topic of interest to you, but it is beyond the scope of this book.

For that reason, when we have had short flirtations with vegetarianism in my house, we tend to eat foods from those cultures where vegetarianism tends to be the regular diet. Indian food abounds with vegetarian choices. So does Middle Eastern food and Ethiopian food. Instead of trying to find substitutes for meat, the recipes are already veggie-based and have been perfected over hundreds of years.

If these dishes aren't to your taste, that's okay, too. The idea of whole food, plant-based eating has been catching on in recent years. The term *plant-based* has been attributed to Thomas Colin Campbell, author of *The China Study*, who first used it in 1980 advocating for a vegan diet. He later began using the term *whole foods* to differentiate the healthy pattern of eating he was promoting from the ultra-processed version of veganism that some who eschew meat had been consuming.[170] There are many physicians, dieticians, and also chefs who are promoting a whole-food, plant-based version of eating, so recipes that focus on real foods abound in books and online, no matter what your food preferences may be.

Cluck That: Considerations with Chicken

I have a cookbook that devotes an entire chapter to what one can make with a rotisserie chicken. I used to love the idea of grabbing a ready-made rotisserie chicken from the supermarket, adding a couple of sides, and voilà—dinner was served! It wasn't fried, and it felt healthy. I thought I was doing the right thing. Until the day I actually read the label on the rotisserie chicken I had quickly grabbed from under the warming kiosk at the supermarket. I was expecting to see chicken and some spices listed. I was not expecting to see modified food starch, carrageenan, and maltodextrin. And yet, there they were.

Why on earth would these items be in my rotisserie chicken? I had previously pictured a supermarket employee preparing the whole unsold chickens from the refrigerator case, putting them on the giant skewers, sprinkling some spices on, and placing them onto the industrial-sized spits in the back. I was sure that I had even witnessed some of these steps while waiting not-so-patiently at the deli counter. And I had. What I hadn't witnessed was when the chickens were being mass-produced for just the purpose of becoming rotisserie chickens, the modified food starch was added to make the skin thicker and crispier and the carrageenan added to help it last longer.[171] Even a local specialty market, which I had wrongly assumed handmade their products from scratch, had opted for these pre-coated chickens. They had a full catering kitchen in back, but the label on the chicken I had picked up revealed that the cooks weren't spending time with the chickens going onto the rotisserie spit. The ingredient label was no different from the one in my grocery store. However, the price was a few dollars higher, again, dispelling the notion that if I spent more for food, I would automatically be getting a better-quality product. The only way I could get an additive-free rotisserie chicken was to purchase one specifically labeled as such at the natural food market and spend twice as much to avoid the additives. I did (and recognize that this is a privilege not everyone has), and after adding some lime and salsa, the chicken was indistinguishable from the ones with additives.

I had to wonder if food producers are so used to using these additives on mass-produced items that they don't even try to season foods the old-fashioned way anymore (some might suggest it is probably cheaper for them to do so and therefore increases their profit margins).

Simple roast chicken is a great, versatile food that's been overly tinkered with. If more consumers start demanding chicken without the additives, its production will become more wide scale and its price will hopefully drop. Until then, if you are able to afford it, remember to read the labels and try to buy chicken that's just chicken.

Processed Meats

While we can make the argument that chicken is healthy, I've yet to see the claim that salted, cured meat is. And yet, only very few of us eat healthy foods all the time. If we are eating a food we know is probably not the best for us, should we just give up completely? Like a dieter who takes a bite of chocolate cake feels they have gone off course, and so continues to eat the entire thing. Does eating a food that is less than perfect mean we should just consume the additive-laden version? I would argue that we shouldn't. We should be eating intuitively and never feel deprived. Deprivation leads to binging.[172] So if you want to eat something, eat it. And if an emulsifier-free version is available and affordable, try to choose that one. Salted, cured meats are enjoyable for me (in moderation!). I enjoyed them in Italy. Could I do the same back home?

While the prepackaged deli meats on display in the refrigerated case contained modified food starches and carrageenan, an internet search of many of my favorite brands of meats on offer at the deli counter contained the mysterious natural flavors but otherwise seemed okay. Salt isn't great for heart disease, and some deli meats have nitrates, which have been linked to various diseases, so deli meat should be a special treat, and the fewer ingredients in them, the better.

Much of the concern over processed meats is due to sulfites. While not an emulsifier and more of a preservative, they're worth a brief mention here. Sulfites, even at levels regarded as safe, can have negative impacts on bacteria in the gut.[173] As a result, the IOIBD has suggested that sufferers of colitis should avoid sulfites.[174] It probably isn't a bad idea for those of us trying to build better microbiomes to do likewise.

Alas, sulfites are common in many processed meat items like bacon, sausage, and encased meats (like salami and pepperoni). No one is arguing these items are healthy for us, but let's face it, they're delicious. And as an occasional side or addition to a sauce, why not? Less processed versions can definitely be found, especially of bacon. Sausage is a little harder to find without the no-no additives but not impossible if you prefer it and are a careful label reader.

Eat Everything Easy Meal Idea: Charcuterie Plate

When we want to get fancy but not really fancy, I make a charcuterie plate. The meat is a small portion of it, and it draws my kids in to get them to eat more fruits and veggies. As much as we all love meat, I try to make it a side, not the main event.

I first did this for my son when he was a toddler. The colors and textures were a big draw and got him eating foods he normally wouldn't. Restaurant professionals say that half of what they do is in the presentation. A good presentation makes ordinary food a little bit special. This one is so easy and actually (potentially) healthy, not to mention delicious.

If I told my kids they were going to eat a bunch of veggie sticks on a plate, it wouldn't happen, but arrange it nicely and place a few bits of meat and cheese on it, and watch it disappear!

Here's how I make a charcuterie plate for two people:

Ingredients

¼ cup cubed cheddar or other additive-free cheese (slice it off a block—if stored properly, a block of hard cheese can last a few weeks in the fridge)

2 slices of Muenster or other sliced cheese (tip: roll up individual slices and then slice vertically every ¼ inch to create pretty party-platter rolls)

2 slices of deli turkey, salami, or meat of your choice, rolled up and sliced as above

10 additive-free crackers, spread out in a fanlike pattern

Carrot sticks, red pepper strips, celery sticks, grapes, apple slices, or whatever fresh veggies or fruit you have on hand, sliced as pretty as you can

If you have them, dried fruits (sulfite-free if you can find it) or nuts make a nice extra component

Steps

1. Lay all ingredients on a platter as fancily as you can. I mentally divide the plate into thirds and arrange the meat and cheese in one part, the crackers in another, and the fruits or veggies in the last one.

2. I yell "charcuterie plate," and everyone comes running. Because my family likes to pretend we're fancy. Yours might too!

Shrimp Can Be a Big Deal (Other Seafood, Too)

It wasn't too long ago that people were told not to eat shrimp owing to their cholesterol content. We were told that this cheap and easy-to-prepare food was bad for our heart. Evidence is now mounting that it isn't the cholesterol content in our food that contributes to our high cholesterol levels.[175] Ultra-processed foods may be more responsible for someone's skyrocketing cholesterol,[176] and whole-food diets that embrace fish, like the Mediterranean diet, have been shown to be particularly healthy, with adherents having lower rates of various chronic diseases.[177] While seafood dishes can be intricate, many simple and delicious seafood dishes can be made in minutes and are a great choice for a quick weeknight meal. (As with other proteins, just check ingredients on packaged premade seafood items.)

Eggs Are Awesome

If you are as old as I am, you may remember when eggs weren't seen as a healthy choice, and egg substitutes abounded. Fake eggs were supposed to be better than the real thing, just like margarine was supposed to be healthier than butter. Spoiler alert: nope. A fill-in-the-blank food substitute is almost certain to contain emulsifiers, thickeners, and other potentially microbiome-disrupting additives to turn what something actually is into something it isn't. Don't fall for this food substitute trap. Go for the real thing every time. And eggs are almost too easy to cook up if you are looking for a quick protein fix and a hot breakfast. They can even be hard-boiled and left in the fridge for days if you need them even more quickly as a grab-and-go item or added to lunch boxes.

So if you feel like indulging in a breakfast sandwich (or anything else), pick the least processed versions of the food you are craving and go for it. Most of my patients wound up quitting diets because they were just too restrictive all the time. Whatever you wind up eating, if you can leave the emulsifiers and fake flavor enhancers out, you're off to a great start. That gets a little bit more challenging when we discuss desserts, but now that you have basic principles for eating less processed foods, we're ready to enjoy the best part of the meal.

Eat Everything Easy Meal Idea: Dawn's Less Processed Egg McFaulkner

For me, the most delicious option for eggs is to incorporate them into a breakfast sandwich. Sometimes a light breakfast is great, but after twenty-four hours on duty as a medical resident in a Boston-area community hospital, I'd march straight down to the cafeteria for my reward: a greasy bacon, egg, and cheese sandwich on an English muffin that we affectionately dubbed the Egg McFaulkner (after the name of the hospital). There was nothing better for what we called being post-call. The seemingly indefatigable man in the chef's hat who prepared them would look at my bedraggled 6 AM appearance, take pity on me, and add six or seven slices of bacon to it. (Don't judge. I'll remind you that the title of this book is *Eat Everything* and not *Eat Healthy All the Time*. There are other books for that, and some of them are very good. But it can make us feel better to indulge when we're having a difficult day.)

Even this splurge breakfast can be made better for us with the right ingredients. The first challenge is procuring English muffins without additives. This has become less of a challenge over the past few years, with natural food markets and Trader Joe's carrying English muffins preserved with vinegar, no other additives, and shoppers accepting a shorter shelf life. Check the labels (this can even be done online from the comfort of your home before you venture out) to find an additive-free brand. Eggs are easy. Cheese, if it comes in a block or even sliced, can be a perfect addition (just avoid the processed cheese singles or the pre-shredded kind). Finally, and thankfully, it's not too hard to find bacon without thickeners and emulsifiers. Try to get sulfite-free versions if you can.

Chapter 9

Desserts

A balanced diet is having a cookie in each hand.
—*Barbara Johnson*

Thomas had tried to quit his dessert habit. He knew that the sweet treats his wife bought for their kids were not helping his waistline. He could give up the cookies and cakes for a week or two, but a visiting cousin, a trip back home, or just a football game might cause him to relapse. And once he went in for the dessert, Thomas went all in, devouring half a bag of cookies or a quarter of a cake in one sitting. He felt like he was somehow addicted to sweets—the more he had, the more he wanted.

He noted he hadn't always reacted this way around desserts. When he was younger, he could have a small portion and walk away. There was something about eating desserts these days that was making him feel like he was never quite satisfied. He always craved more. So Thomas had decided that the most sensible thing for him to do was to avoid desserts altogether (though he wasn't always successful attaining this goal).

In his book, *Hooked*, the journalist Michael Moss lays out a compelling argument for how we become addicted to certain foods, especially sweets. Basically, when certain substances hit our brain fast, we get a high-like experience, and sugar can send signals from our tongue to our brain in seconds.[178] So vulnerable individuals will crave sugar. We want that high.

That explains a lot, but it doesn't explain why so many of us like Thomas never seem to be satisfied when eating modern ultra-processed foods. For this, we have to keep reading. Moss goes on to describe an experiment where participants are offered two glasses of water, one plain and one with the additive maltodextrin used. It is used as an additive in many sweets, as discussed in earlier chapters of this book, but turns out to be not so sweet on its own.[179] When asked to pick the better water, most of the participants picked the maltodextrin-containing one. Moss attributes this to the excess calories in the maltodextrin, causing our GI system to send signals of approval to our brain.

So Thomas had rightly concluded that he had an addiction to ultra-processed desserts—one that he developed later in life, since he hadn't had that problem earlier. Had the desserts changed, had his microbiome changed, or was it the former perhaps leading to the latter? Thomas didn't want to give up dessert entirely, but he wanted to be able to stop eating sweets when he was satisfied. Could he do that with real desserts? He decided to give it a try but, as he soon discovered, finding premade desserts made without additives can be challenging.

Enjoying Some Sweet Treats

No Italian meal (or American meal, for that matter) would be complete without dessert. Besides gelato and a wide variety of cookies and cakes, the Italians have brought the world tiramisu—the holy trinity of desserts—combining cake, cream, and coffee in one dish. The hallmark of Italian desserts (in Italy) is their freshness. Cannoli shells are fried that day. Cream is whipped that hour. You can smell the intoxicating egg, flour, and sugar combinations melding together when walking past bakeries in any Italian city or town. And like the artichoke hawkers, the bakers want you to witness the process of creation, rolling out their doughs in front of large plate glass windows.

The tastes are subtle. Instead of being overwhelmed by sweetness, you are entranced by creaminess and depth of flavor. Whole pistachio nuts alight on top of cookies, and fresh fruits decorate cakes. These desserts are truly spectacular. But most of us can't go to our neighborhood supermarket to pick up anything like an Italian dessert. Desserts at most grocery stores are mass-produced off-site

Homemade and Ultra-Processed

Until recently, it could be assumed that if you were making food in your own home, it would not be ultra-processed. Now, at least in the US, industrial-grade ingredients are available on your grocery shelf—sometimes even, and especially, on the shelves of health food stores.

In the twenty-first century, xanthan gum has made its way into many gluten-free pantries as an alternative binding agent to gluten.[180] It is generally available next to whole grain flours in health food stores, giving us the illusion that it is promoting wellness. The next several years may see other industrial additives making their way onto supermarket shelves for home cooks to experiment with.

and made to withstand transportation and storage for long periods of time. Some desserts are baked on-site at grocery stores, but like fast-casual sandwich shops, only the last step may be completed at the grocery bakery.

Scratch bakeries can be found, but they are rare. While baking one cake or a tray of cookies isn't at all difficult (trust me, you can bake), baking in large quantities, if not done in a factory, requires a lot of equipment and hands. And baked goods don't have large profit margins—maybe a few dollars on a cake and a few quarters on a cookie. Being a baker isn't a terribly secure business in the US. The mass-produced cakes and cookies undercut the local handmade stuff every time.

Thomas was trying to improve his cholesterol and sugar numbers, but some people struggling with bowel symptoms feel as if they have to give up dessert altogether even if their blood work is perfect. They notice that more than anything else, skipping dessert helps reduce their GI upset post-meal. And looking at the ingredient list on a store-bought cake, it's easy to see why.

The list could be a glossary of additives that potentially lead to gastrointestinal upset: mono- and diglycerides, polysorbate 60 or 80, modified food starch, soy lecithin, and not one but three types of food gums—cellulose, guar, and xanthan in just one cake! Even the cakes sold at natural food markets or high-end grocery stores contain many, if not all, of these ingredients. A trip to my nearest US-based Italian market provided little better. Sadly, these bakeries were seemingly Italian in name only.

How to Build a Better Dessert

I'm not suggesting that we give up on sweet treats to end our meals. I'm proposing that we turn down giant servings of cheaply produced, indefinitely preserved, and average-tasting baked goods in favor of small, sensible portions of the really good stuff.

If lacking a real bakery nearby or sufficient funds to support a regular real bakery habit, we have to consider trying to make desserts ourselves. This may actually be a pretty good idea. In his book *Cooked*, Michael Pollan quotes food and diet expert Harry Balzer and suggests we can have any decadent food item we want, but we have to make it ourselves, therefore limiting the quantity of dessert we can consume.[181] If you want cake and brownies and tiramisu, no problem. Make it. While making our own bread or pasta is not realistic for most, making the occasional sweet treat may be. And though it will cost us some time, it could be argued that this may be a great way to self-regulate our intake of sweets.

I'd be remiss as a physician if I didn't add that we should be attempting to limit or even avoid added sugars completely. There. I said it. And we should. But we are human, and we like sugar. So go on and have a little. Like butter or salt, sugar is a Group 2 food in the Nova classification system—it is an indulgence and mainly meant as an accompaniment to enhance whole Group 1 foods.

The extent to which added sugar, salt, and fat have been dumped into ultra-processed foods has had the perverse effect of home cooks abandoning those ingredients, that, let's face it, make food taste good. So people who would otherwise be competent home cooks instead wind up buying ultra-processed foods that are far worse for our health than adding sugar to homemade dishes would be.

Many of the ingredients that plague store-bought confections can be found in cake mixes, brownie mixes, and ready-to-bake cookie doughs, too. Food gums abound in cake mixes, carrageenan can be found in brownie mixes, and soy lecithin is in cookie dough. Add a little frosting from a small shelf-stable tub and you're now eating polysorbate 60. Unfortunately, the ingredients in mixes are much less like anything actually homemade and are basically the same stuff that's in the grocery cakes. And those ingredients are totally unnecessary. You can easily bake a cake without them. It's just generations of marketing that have led you to think that you need a mix.

The boxed mixes were introduced in the 1930s and really took off in the 1950s, when food looking as unnatural as possible seems to have had its heyday. Add a few eggs, oil, and water, and voilà—cake! But unlike the popular mid-century Jell-O molds and everything-as-a-casserole concoctions, cake mixes and their frosting tub partners seem to have had staying power. When people said in the 1990s that they baked from scratch, this meant they were using mixes at home.[182]

But DIY-ing cakes, cookies, and brownies isn't at all hard. There's no painstaking kneading or rolling or cutting to be done. There's no timing dough rising just right. Actually, baking simple desserts from scratch turns out to be exactly like baking from a mix, except for remembering to take out a stick of butter and some eggs in advance to bring them up to room temperature (if you forget to do this, no problem: find a large glass, fill it with boiling water, let it sit for ten to twenty seconds, and then pour the water out. Invert the glass over the stick of butter or egg, and in a couple of minutes it will be up to room temperature, or close enough). You'll have to pull out a few more containers than just one box—flour, sugar, baking soda or powder, and maybe some cocoa and vanilla extract—and add a couple of measuring cups and spoons to the kitchen counter, but that only takes a few more minutes. If we are being honest, the real problem is the increase in dishes home-baking desserts creates. But loved ones are easily bribed with brownies to take on the dish washing.

While we are on the topic of indulging, it may be the right time to talk about drinks.

Chapter 10

Drinks

I would rather suffer with coffee than be senseless.

—Napoleon Bonaparte

The to-go cup has in recent years become a symbol of the harried American. And perhaps no one exemplifies the harried American more than my long-established patient Martha who one day came to see me for a regular checkup. Martha is a forty-five-year-old coffee lover. I have rarely seen her without a to-go cup in her hand. I call up Martha's history on my computer screen while her clear plastic cup starts to sweat onto my desk. Today, her cup is filled with a gloppy, semi-frozen, colorful concoction without much resemblance to coffee. I have to ask.

"What is *that*?" I say, pointing at the drink—forgetting for a moment to be nonjudgmental.

Martha laughs. She explains that her teenage daughter wanted one, so she got one for herself, too. It's a new drink being offered by her favorite chain coffee shop. "It's horrible," she admits. "I'm not sure why I gave in and bought it. I should probably throw the rest out. It definitely isn't agreeing with me."

"What do you mean?" I ask.

Martha went on to confide that it wasn't just the colorful not-coffee drink but many different foods and drinks that had been giving her trouble for the past few months. She was spending a lot more time in the bathroom than she used to.

"Is it perimenopause?" she asked.

"Maybe," I said. "Have you changed anything in your diet?"

Martha confided that she hadn't, though she had been eating fairly unhealthily the past few years. Divorced with three kids, two heavily involved in sports, it seemed as if she spent half her life in the car. Most days she was able to work from home but found she didn't have time to cook. In the evenings, she'd swing by drive-throughs on her way home from one activity or another, and when there wasn't even time for that, meal delivery services provided the dinner solution. Pizza, burritos, and rotisserie chicken were her main dinner staples. Drinks from the coffee shop fueled her morning after dropping the kids off at two different schools, with a second serving on many afternoons. She had switched to soy or almond milk because she had heard these were healthier and might be easier on her GI system, but that didn't seem to help much. Or at all. Still, as busy as she was, and as guilty as she was about the relative unhealthiness of the rest of her diet, Martha continued to get her drinks with milk alternatives. She figured it was better than doing nothing.

I had to let her down gently that it probably wasn't any better and quite possibly worse. In fact, many popular beverages (from our flavored coffees to bottled sodas and juices) contain additives that we need to be aware of if we want a happier microbiome and better health.

The Stuff in Milk Alternatives

Martha was ordering nondairy milks thinking they'd be better for her. Of course, part of the trouble of ordering a drink at a coffee shop is that (unless you're grabbing a premade one from the to-go cooler) it won't come with an ingredient list. A quick google search revealed that along with the almonds (which would be just fine, since she didn't have a nut allergy), she was often downing lecithin, guar gum, and xanthan gum with her afternoon coffee beverage. The soy milk she occasionally also ordered contained carrageenan. Most commercially available milk alternatives are made with emulsifiers to keep them smooth and mixed. Unless you are making the alternative milk in your own kitchen or buying from a specialty shop that guarantees it grinds its nut milks itself, odds are that you are downing a lot of additives with your java. Likewise, for the coffee creamers.

So what's a coffee lover to do? Lactose-free milk is rarely available in coffee shops, so if you think you suffer from lactose intolerance (but have not actually been formally diagnosed) and are trying to avoid milk but also trying to avoid food additives, I suggest performing your own experiment. In Italy, if you order a cappuccino, it will probably contain an ounce or two of espresso and not more than four ounces of milk. Often people who have some lactose intolerance can tolerate small amounts of dairy, just as William from chapter 5 discovered he could. Try the smallest coffee drink you can, preferably less than six ounces, made with real milk Italian-style. Or drink plain drip coffee or an Americano (espresso and water) with just a splash of milk.

Artificial Sweeteners

Unless you have diabetes, use real sugar as a sweetener (but just a bit—remember what we talked about in chapter 9!). Or add honey (still, just a little). Avoid the calorie-free alternative sweeteners, which are another potential source of bowel distress.

The most popular sweetener today might be sucralose, usually found in a yellow packet. Sucralose is a short-chain sugar with a bond that our bodies cannot digest. As a result, it can cause bloating, diarrhea, and gas. Another alternative sweetener that has boldly declared itself as being natural and therefore markets itself as better, is stevia, usually in a greenish packet. Unfortunately, stevia is yet another carbohydrate that our intestines cannot break down (anything that has no calories means your body can't break it down as it would actual food). Additionally, most commercially available brands include a polyol that the body can struggle with as well and that IBS sufferers have correctly been told to avoid in the low-FODMAP diet. There are other alternative sweeteners out there, but nothing digests as quickly and as easily as real sugar (which poses a problem for those suffering from diabetes, but using sugar in small amounts is probably the best option for nearly everyone else).

Sports Drinks, Premade Iced Teas, and More: Just What's in That Bottle?

I've learned to start being skeptical when something in a package is labeled as a healthy choice. Anything that comes from a package probably isn't that healthy.

In step with this line of thinking, many schools have removed carbonated sodas from their vending machines, touting colorful sports drinks as a healthier alternative. A quick search of the ingredients on the plastic bottle reveals food gums or modified food starches, keeping the bright colors and sugary flavors conveniently mixed for months or maybe years. Bottled iced teas can contain maltodextrin and more gums. Many health shakes, yogurt drinks, and all manner of liquid concoctions contain the panoply of emulsifiers and stabilizers that may be causing trouble for diet-related disease sufferers. It is far less likely that real fruit or yogurt is the problem. It's the extra stuff we are putting in that shouldn't be there in the first place. We are making even healthy food problematic.

Besides containing emulsifiers and stabilizers, many of the prepackaged drinks we consume are sweetened with high-fructose corn syrup. This additive has been maligned for a plethora of health reasons, including diabetes and colon cancer.[183] But could it also play a role in IBS symptoms? People can digest fructose, but not everyone can digest it in high doses. Anywhere from five to fifty grams of it may be too much for some people. At the upper end of consumption, a majority of people have bloating, gas, and diarrhea.[184]

Juices (which contain naturally occurring fructose) and sodas (which have the added fructose) don't have the sugar encased in fiber as it is in whole fruit, to slow down the rush of fructose to the intestines, perhaps resulting in the aforementioned symptoms. A liter of these beverages can have upward of sixty grams of fructose.[185] While, hopefully, not too many of us consume a whole liter in a sitting, a typical bottle is easily half a liter, and that may be enough to upset some stomachs.

What about regular corn syrup? Corn syrup is not the same thing as high-fructose corn syrup. Fructose has to be broken down by the gut before it can be absorbed. If it isn't broken down and travels through the gut intact, it can lead to diarrhea. Again, this is why some people get diarrhea after drinking large quantities of juice or soda—it's the fructose overwhelming the system. Regular corn syrup is basically glucose, not fructose, and glucose is simple enough for the body to absorb without first needing to do anything else to it. Dextrose, another commonly found additive, is a type of glucose, or for the sake of simplicity it essentially is glucose, and is quickly absorbed by the body. While large doses of glucose can cause spikes in blood sugar (this is what pregnant women are given to drink to check for pregnancy-induced diabetes), it is absorbed quickly from the gastrointestinal tract and is therefore not a culprit implicated in IBS symptoms.

So avoiding high-fructose corn syrup, at least in any significant quantities, makes sense for those trying to cope with gastrointestinal distress. It should go without saying (but I'll say it again) that we should limit all sugars in our diet for myriad health reasons—even if glucose and dextrose aren't implicated in bowel troubles. That doesn't mean you can't have anything sweet, but limiting sweet drinks is a pretty good place to start if you are troubled by weight gain or have been told that your blood sugar is in the diabetes or prediabetes range. Can you have a sweet tea or other sweet beverage from time to time? Sure! But from a health perspective, no one should have a sixteen-ounce cloyingly sweet anything on a daily basis.

What About Alcohol?

I was discussing with a gastroenterologist friend whether people who stayed at home during the COVID-19 pandemic had experienced more or fewer GI symptoms while in lockdown. We both agreed that when our patients cooked more, it seemed to help. And then she said something I hadn't expected: she noticed that many of her patients who used to go out drinking felt much better now that they were staying at home.

Sure, many of us feel horrible after a night of overindulging. That's not news. What struck me as odd was that she described an improvement of bowel symptoms I had never associated with alcohol. I wondered what it was besides the alcohol that the patients might have been eliminating when they were forced to stay in. But I wasn't able to find out.

Unlike any other food or drink, alcoholic beverages need not list their ingredients—not on their packaging and not on the makers' websites. This includes drinks that clearly contain sugar, sugar substitutes, creamers, and in all likelihood a whole bunch of emulsifiers and other additives. It turns out that the FDA, as imperfect as it is, has almost no jurisdiction over alcohol. As a remnant of prohibition, alcohol was regulated by the Bureau of Alcohol, Tobacco, Firearms and Explosives (ATF) until 2003 and was only asked to consult with FDA regarding its policies on alcohol.[186] In 2003, a new agency was formed called the Alcohol and Tobacco Tax and Trade Bureau (TTB). According to the TTB, "Our staff is highly educated and technically trained; more than half are analysts, chemists, investigators and auditors. In addition, a large number of employees serve as financial, legal, information management, and computer specialists."[187] They don't seem to have a lot of dieticians on staff.

Makers of alcoholic beverages are merely instructed that they may not use "substances prohibited from use in human food" and they can use anything FDA lists as GRAS,[188] which as reviewed previously, may not be so great for all of us. And they aren't required to tell us about any of their ingredients or additives, save one. The exception to this is sulfites, which you may have seen noted on your wine label (and which you may remember from their brief mention in chapter 8). These are added to food as a preservative meant to impede the growth of bacteria. It's added to wine for the same reason, to help keep it from going off.

Over the years, rare allergic reactions to sulfites have been reported,[189] so in 1986, the FDA ordered that food and drinks contain a label to warn those susceptible to this reaction.[190] Since ATF follows FDA guidance regarding warning labels, this made it onto alcohol labels, too. But don't expect a full list of ingredients to make it onto your alcoholic beverage any time soon. Consumer groups have been asking for this since the 1970s and have been rebuffed every time the issue has come up.[191] It seems food and beverage makers much prefer us not knowing what's in their products.

So what can we do if we are trying to avoid emulsifiers and thickeners? The first thing to do is skip the mixers and flavored alcohols. Might some of them be okay? Sure. But right now there's just no way to know. If you've noticed that beer or wine upsets your system, stick with plain spirits. Maltodextrin can be used by beer makers as a flavor additive. It turns out that acacia gum (also called gum arabic) is used by beer and wine makers to help keep their products looking clear, and in the case of beer make the foam look prettier.[192] Anecdotally, people tell me that wine in Italy or other places doesn't bother them, but wine in the US does. Is it the sulfites? Could it be the food gums? Something else? I don't know because without ingredient labels, we just have no idea what we are consuming. That's really a shame because when we are able to access ingredient labels, we might be able to comfortably eat foods we had previously thought were off-limits.

As a quick reminder, being able to remove something from the off-limits list doesn't mean it can be placed on the no-limits list. Alcohol in large quantities is a poison. It can contribute to gut inflammation and liver inflammation all on its own—no additives required. It has been linked to an increased risk of several cancers.[193] Alcohol isn't healthy, and some people may want to, or need to, avoid it altogether. Yet small amounts of alcohol are considered to be part of the famed Mediterranean diet, and, well, it can be fun. While alcohol is not a health drink, it can be something some of us may want to enjoy on occasion, and we should be able to do that without additives.

What Can We Drink?

We really should try to break our sweet drink habits if we can. The biggest difference my patients with blood sugar issues have seen is when they are able to cut these out. Whether a sports drink, energy drink, or overly sweetened coffee-like beverage, there's not much good going on there. Sure, eat everything, but try to stick to drinking more water or fizzy water during the day.

There's still plenty we can enjoy. If you like tea or coffee (and the coffee doesn't move your bowels too much), they are great hot or iced, but just be careful what you put into them. If you like a little something sweet to drink, coconut water or a lemonade or orange juice that you've made yourself is probably best. If you are drinking something off the shelf, don't buy light versions of the drink—they will have sugar substitutes in them that can cause all kinds of trouble.

Start slowly diluting sugary lemonade or sweet tea with water. If you are used to overly sweetened drinks, it may take a little while but people can usually still enjoy sweet drinks that are half water. That might still be too much for those with blood sugar issues, so be careful. And if you like fermented foods, kombucha and kefir are incredibly tasty. If you've decided alcohol (in moderation) is right for you, then you can also enjoy wine, beer, or a homemade cocktail—hold the premade mixers.

As for sodas, sports drinks, and energy drinks? If you really want one, go for it. But remember that they are a treat and shouldn't be a staple in your diet.

Mainly, if you have a diet-related disease and maybe even if you don't, avoid the complicated drinks and stick to the simple stuff. You can still have good drinks, but try to keep the additives out. If you can do that, you're ready to tackle the broad category of processed foods.

Chapter 11

Processed Foods

It's time to embrace and celebrate ketchup, not be ashamed of it.

—*José Andrés*

If you have a child who plays sports, you might be familiar with being assigned snack duty—bringing snacks for the kids to enjoy after the game. They usually consist of something the team loves like cheese curls or barbeque chips or some kind of cookies in a small aluminum-lined bag. I knew my assignment, yet I wanted to do something different.

"How about we bring a bag of clementines?" I asked my daughter.

"Mom," she responded in the exasperated voice belonging uniquely to tween-aged girls. "Do you *actually* want people to hate us?"

I had to admit I did not.

Scouring the supermarket shelves for something that would be palatable to the kids but not make me feel like I was promoting unhealthy snacking, I was reminded of the bambini boxes on Italian trains known as Trenitalia.

What Trenitalia lacks in punctuality, it definitely makes up for in the quality and presentation of its snacks. To my kids' great surprise and enjoyment, while the adults were offered freshly made espresso and our choice of a sweet or a savory snack, the kids were given colorful cardboard boxes to open. What McDonald's figured out a long time ago and what all parents learn by our children's second birthday is that opening a box makes what's inside all the more exciting. In Italy, my kids joyfully tore into their boxes and found an activity page with crayons, a small bottle of water, and both a sweet and a savory snack bag. The snacks were simple potato chips and chocolate butter cookies. No wild colors, no flavor enhancers. There were only a handful of ingredients listed on each of the packages. No one was pretending this was health food, but I didn't feel terrible that my kids were eating it. And if I'm being honest, the cookies were a big hit with the kids (and the adults who had opted for the sweet snack), whereas the chips were rated as just okay. I wondered if Italian kids, not raised on unnaturally red, flaming-hot cheese curls, would have liked the chips better than my kids did.

By way of an answer, my son showed me a YouTube video after we had returned to the US. It featured young Italians trying American snacks and being mostly horrified. Upon looking at the packaging, one woman expressed her doubt about American ingredients. Another tried to explain to his presumed American audience that we should be aware that there are better things to eat. Finally, one young man suggested he was wary of visiting the US after partaking of the things we snack on.[194]

Ultimately, I decided that Italian kids probably do like plain chips a lot more than my American kids. Not because there is something inherently different about kids raised on either side of the Atlantic Ocean, but because we become accustomed to what we eat, and we have become used to increasingly ultra-processed foods. Remember, according to the Nova food classification system, there's a big difference between processed and ultra-processed, though people use these terms interchangeably quite often. Processed foods may not be so bad for us, unlike the ultra-processed versions of something similar. I'm not trying to propose that chips are health food, only that we can enjoy less processed versions of foods that are not being eaten for their nutritional value.

US children, and their parents, have been raised on a steady diet of food that no longer resembles actual food. Simple crackers and chips given to toddlers are soon overtaken by their increasingly ultra-processed brethren by the time the kids are in elementary school. Packaged food purveyors are constantly trying to get our attention, so they add more flashiness and flavors to their wares. And then even that's not enough. Like the cardboard boxes my kids got to open on Trenitalia, we like a little surprise with our snacks. Snacking isn't a time to eat serious food. It has evolved into a time for fun food. So in an effort to continue to surprise and delight, the food industry has been raising the bar on snacks' wow factor year after year.

Bags of chips line shelves for nearly an entire aisle in my supermarket. Colors have gone neon, fire appears to jump from the label, and promises of more flavor are made. But how, exactly, are we getting all that flavor?

Sweetness and Spice, but Not Too Nice

Maltodextrin seems to find its way to the beginning of ingredient lists on snack foods, sometimes listed as the third or fourth ingredient in a dizzyingly long list. As a reminder, maltodextrin is a long-chain sugar that the human gut can digest, and it does so relatively quickly. It has been suspected of altering the gut microbiome and potentially causing inflammation and perhaps even contributing to the development of IBD like Crohn's.[195] Maltodextrin is found even in snack foods from natural food markets because it is often derived from foods such as corn, so it's considered natural (again, beware of this marketing word). It imparts a certain sweetness to foods while also enhancing other flavors. Maltodextrin is probably the most difficult additive to avoid in snack foods, but given its potential effects on the gut, you should try to.

Which brings us back to the snack aisle and what the heck I'm going to bring to the soccer game. Like the train attendant, I first have to ask, sweet or savory? That question doesn't matter so much, according to my daughter. Kids like both. So do adults.

If I go the savory route, I could choose from chips, popcorn, pretzels, or some kind of veggie- or cheese-flavored sticks. Though the flavor options read Barbeque, Chili, or Ranch, in my mind I see *Maltodextrin* instead. Or I could go with plain. It turns out that many versions of ordinary potato chips have just potato, oil, and salt. The same goes for tortilla or pita chips. Plain pretzels are just wheat and salt. Salted popcorn is sometimes okay, too. I have to read the labels, but there are actually several options if I was happy with just salt as a flavoring.

Do you want them to hate us? I hear my daughter's question echoing in the back of my mind.

Mild dislike might be okay, I reason as I make my way to the sweets aisle. There, the equally colorful cookie packages declare they contain real chocolate or they are made with whole grains. I wonder if going sweet might be the better option—perhaps pairing fewer additives with less tween angst? Turns out, no. Maltodextrin is still ubiquitous on these ingredient lists. Also, soy lecithin is in nearly everything.

And then there is polysorbate 60 and polysorbate 80. Polysorbate is another emulsifier, and it's made by combining a fatty acid with a polyol. It's used to make chocolate or frostings smoother. It's also used in some bread products as a dough conditioner and in powdered mixes as a dispersing agent.[196] While in small doses it has been deemed not to be a cancer-causing agent or a substance that could cause reproductive issues, it has been seen in animal studies to cause diarrhea in repeat-dose toxicity studies.[197]

As with studies of many other additives, human studies of polysorbate have been limited, with no more than a couple of dozen participants studied for a week or two at most. A similarly small number of infants have been studied for slightly longer periods of time,[198] but it is difficult to ask infants to assess if they feel differently while ingesting a different diet. They complain a lot as it is. Most disturbingly, scientists have found that polysorbate can make the gut more susceptible to the movement of *E. coli* bacteria across the cellular barrier of the intestinal tract, perhaps triggering an inflammatory response in susceptible individuals. It has been implicated in the possible development of Crohn's disease.[199] So research is pointing to polysorbate causing stomach upset in some and potentially life-threatening colitis in others. I cannot think of one good reason to consume this additive.

Likewise with titanium dioxide. As of May 2021, the EFSA, which is re-examining the data around many food additives, decided to decertify titanium dioxide as a food additive, declaring it is "no longer considered safe." The EFSA pointed to studies suggesting that nanoparticles of titanium dioxide could accumulate in cells, alter DNA, and potentially have cancer-causing effects.[200] Meanwhile, due to the inflammatory effects seen in the guts of people with colitis, the IOIBD cautioned both Crohn's disease and UC sufferers to avoid this additive.[201] I think that's probably enough for us all to stay away from titanium dioxide as a food additive, where it is mainly used to make things like marshmallows and frostings whiter. If a treat you are about to eat has something blindingly white on or in it, pay particular attention to the label.

Lastly, glycerin appears on some cookie ingredient lists. This ingredient rings a bell. First, because it is the title of a rock song popular in the 1990s. Second, because glycerin suppositories are used in medicine to induce a bowel movement. It draws water into the colon in constipated patients, which helps the stool move out. But the cookies are going in the other way. Need I worry? It turns out that glycerin is the same as glycerol, another polyol that IBS patients are supposed to avoid. It is also used to soothe oral irritation, but users are supposed to take caution not to swallow excessive amounts of it.[202] While there probably aren't massive amounts of glycerin being used to make cookies softer and sweeter, I think I better avoid glycerin, too. This ingredient isn't used in hard cookies without fillings, so it's easy enough to skip.

I now have a decision to make, but instead of sweet or savory, it is maltodextrin or polysorbate. Neither sounds great.

And then I remember. Not being able to eat these ingredients is my problem. I'm not on a crusade to take tasty snacks away from American children or to be a food scold. But if we are being honest, making snacking healthier for everyone wouldn't be a bad thing.

To that end, I compromise. I decide that I won't provide snacks with additives that have been implicated in possibly inducing colitis in susceptible people, but I won't be as strict with additives as I am with my usual grocery shopping. I go with plain pretzels (perhaps inducing mild disappointment) and small candy bars (doubtlessly making up for my other, blander choice). The kids are, as far as I know, without gastrointestinal complaints or blood sugar troubles. In all likelihood, they can partake of the candy and suffer no ill effects. I do, however, grab that bag of clementines. You never know what kids might go for.

Just kidding. We totally know what kids go for. I end up eating them.

I am not going to convince kids raised on a diet of intense marketing and intense artificial flavors to change their habits overnight—my son is more likely than not to pick up a bag of flaming-hot cheese curls when he stops at a convenience store with his friends. But I've made it a point to stock up on less processed versions of processed foods in the hopes that when the teen years are done, examples for healthier eating will have been internalized.

Using Processed Foods to Make Less Processed Meals

If we have the privilege of time and money and are able to prepare foods at home, how do we not fall into the trap of using ultra-processed foods in our own kitchens? For many of us, the reality of weeknight food preparation can be generously described as barely contained chaos. There's a reason cooking videos are sped up and visually beautiful. There probably isn't a huge market for people wanting to watch food preparation in the context of multiple small children running around, one of whom has been offended to the point of funeral tears by another, while something else overcooks on the stove.

In general, even on our weekends, we are overburdened, overworked, and overscheduled. We are tired. We don't need more to do, we need less. We can't be expected to be scratch cooks every night or even most of them. Harried home cooks have to use shortcuts—sauces, dressings, marinades, and the like. There is no way to get dinner on the table in thirty minutes without them (and that's often a generous allotment for the busy, tired, and overworked). The problem is that cooking shortcuts are often fraught with additive booby traps. The good news is that not all of them are, and there are work-arounds to the old standbys that make getting food on the table fast while avoiding the drivers of diet-related disease.

Better Sauces, Mixes, and Marinades—DIY or Don't!

Let's consider those wax-coated cardboard boxes of stocks, broths, and bouillon cubes as a quick flavoring fix. The first time I cooked couscous with chicken broth instead of water, I was ready to crown myself top chef only to later discover that real chefs hire a kitchen assistant called a saucier, whose only job is to make stocks from scratch. So along with freshly baking bread and handcrafting pasta, please add stock making to the list of things we mostly do not have time for. And let's be honest, the premade broths do the trick. Some of them contain food gums and maltodextrin. Happily, plenty of brands available at a regular grocery store do not. These brands are often just as good, if not better. Check the label and then use your preferred brand liberally to add restaurant-level flavor.

Sauces and marinades can be made from scratch fairly quickly. The key is to pair an acid with a fat and throw in some salt, garlic, or other spices. So lemon juice and olive oil plus a little salt, pepper, and garlic; or lime, sesame oil, and soy

Prepare for Battle

Having the tools to make chopping less of a chore or squeezing lemons in seconds can also make food preparation a reasonable activity to try to undertake. Here are some tools that I've found useful:

- Handheld citrus press, $15
- Garlic press, $10–$15
- Good-quality peeler (if you have a bad peeler, it can take twice as long), $10
- Good-quality box grater (again, a bad one will cost you time), $15
- Dicer or chopper (you don't need to splurge on this if you're handy with a knife), $25
- Good chef's knife (you do need this as it saves time and fingertips), $20–$$$

Pressure cookers and slow cookers can also be valuable kitchen additions to help cut down on mealtime chaos. You don't need them or have to spend a lot here. And you don't need to get all of these items at once. Start cooking and considering where you might need to shave some time off your food preparation.

sauce, plus garlic and ginger. You can get incredibly creative or you can google ideas (or you can look at the end of this book). Or if pressed for time, you can open a bottle of something. There are great Asian-style marinades, amazing barbeque sauces, and all kinds of ideas on your grocery store shelves for throwing together a quick meal. But just like dressings, these can contain myriad emulsifiers and thickeners like gums and modified starches. Some brands do, and, thankfully, some brands don't.

The next crutch even the best home cooks have come to rely on is premixed spice packets or jars. Like the rotisserie chicken and the broth, how on earth could commercial food purveyors manage to mess this one up? Just take some spices and add them to a packet, right? Well, not usually. Oftentimes there is maltodextrin and other agents added. While ostensibly included to reduce clumping of the powder, given the cost of some spices, adding these agents bulks them up so that the overall cost to produce them goes down. Thankfully, the cost of making your own spice mixes and rubs is definitely cheaper than buying them, and as an added bonus, they're additive-free.

A simple rub for meat can be made by adding your favorite dried herbs to some sea salt. A Tex-Mex mix for fajitas or taco nights is salt, paprika, cumin, garlic, oregano, and a little chili pepper if you are in the mood. Mix a container full of the stuff when you have an extra five minutes and grab it from the pantry when you need it.

It sounds pretty easy, but I'm not going to lie to you. Getting into the rhythm of additive-free cooking does take some time. The makers of all the foods we have come to rely on, even if we pride ourselves on being decent home cooks, have spent a lot of money trying to convince us that we need them. Learning a new way of cooking presents initial hurdles, but these can be overcome in a matter of weeks of careful label reading.

Buying some additive-free staples to have on hand, if you use them a lot, can save an incredible amount of time. If you have friends or family members who cook, ask them what they do. People who cook a lot generally have some tricks to share. Or maybe join a cooking group on social media. You'll find there are different strategies, but one may be the lightbulb idea that helps you shave off a few minutes here and there and makes it more likely you'll be able to make additive-free meals.

For example, some may use a garlic press, while others may keep a jar of crushed garlic in their fridge. Friends have taught me to find a few minutes to mince fresh garlic and ginger and then freeze them in baggies or in an ice tray to use later. You can get minced garlic and even frozen ginger packets from the grocery store. While this isn't exactly at the same level of professional food preparers on television shows, having stuff ready to go can make a big difference.

The Lowdown on Condiments

Ketchup, mustard, and mayonnaise are the trifecta of spreads and the base for a lot of sauces and dressings, so getting these right can make a big difference.

Ketchup is a quintessentially American food invented in the late 1800s, a time that might be considered the dawn of the modern processed food era. While John Harvey Kellogg was pondering ways to make breakfast less sexually appealing for his health spa patients,[203] Henry John Heinz was pushing back—inventing condiments to spice up plain American food. His biggest success was Heinz Tomato Ketchup.[204]

Heinz was known as a strong proponent of a movement focused on food purity and worker safety, helping to usher in the Pure Food and Drug Act of 1906.[205] Heinz went through many iterations of the ketchup until he could figure out how to make it additive-free. According to the Heinz archives, the recipe in 1895 called for tomatoes; a hearty mix of spices such as cloves, cinnamon, garlic, and onion; vinegar; sugar; and salt.[206] I suspect it was delicious.

Unfortunately, I'm not quite sure that Henry Heinz would be pleased with what he would find in today's US supermarkets: standard ketchup contains high-fructose corn syrup and "natural flavoring" to replace some of the more than half-dozen spices originally used. There are, however, natural and simple versions that don't contain high-fructose corn syrup and are closest to the preparation most commonly found on supermarket shelves in Europe.

Avoiding ketchup with additives isn't terribly difficult once you start looking at labels, and it isn't difficult to avoid other condiments with additives, either. Mustard, ketchup's trusty sidekick, can be a versatile ingredient. Traditional yellow mustard is made with mustard seed, vinegar, and spices. But modified food starch can find its way onto the ingredient lists. Dijon mustard substitutes wine or wine vinegar for the regular vinegar and often leaves out the modified starches and extra flavorings. Brown mustards are another good alternative, but, as always, check the ingredient lists.

Mayonnaise is the third part of our trifecta. Perhaps because of its high fat content (it's made primarily of oil and eggs), mayo can get a bad rap. Not too long ago, the medical establishment had (incorrectly) declared fat the enemy. So in a performative effort at healthfulness, the food industry began to remove it from processed foods—including from much of our mayo.

When you remove a substance, especially one as much beloved by the human tongue as fat, you need to replace it with something—something that our body doesn't recognize as fat and can't digest and use as a form of energy (so it's also low-calorie). Enter, again, modified food starches and gums. The top three ingredients of Hellmann's Real Mayonnaise, for example, are oil, water, and eggs/egg yolks. For its light mayo, though, the top three ingredients are water, oil, and

Emulsification—Separating the Good From the Bad

Mayonnaise is an emulsification—a substance created by the combining of oil and water that otherwise wouldn't want to mix and stay mixed. The protein in the egg helps the oil and water molecules combine and stay that way, at least for a while. Mixing at high speeds and/or heating ingredients in a specific order creates a little chemistry lab, resulting in creamy sauces and dressings when done properly. But natural emulsifications won't stay together forever unless there is something in the mixture that creates strong bonds between the oil and water components. That's where a lot of the food additives that have been discussed in this book come in. Food purveyors will add emulsifiers, like the gums, to all kinds of products to make them hold together and stay attractive on the shelf for months or even years.

modified food starch. The additive has now virtually become the food, meaning that in our quest for low-fat or reduced-calorie healthfulness, some of us are consuming greater amounts of nonfood ingredients than regulators had initially accounted for. Remember, at high enough levels, nonabsorbable food items bring GI distress to anyone. It is probably a good idea for all of us to avoid low-fat options of foods that are basically supposed to be fat. Eat the real thing! Fat is not the enemy. Try to find mayo brands that stick as closely as possible to the real-food ingredients oil, egg, mustard, vinegar, and lemon juice.

In general, for spreads and dips, don't waste your money on fancy labels. Instead, read the ingredient lists carefully, and keep them full-fat.

***

Shake off the idea that all food is processed and there's nothing you can do to improve upon what you are eating. You can make real food, and you can make it really well. Or you can choose to eat out (the next part of the book will give some tips about this). Remember that real food is not the enemy, and neither is processed food.

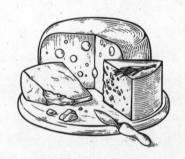

Part III

Eating Everything in Real Life

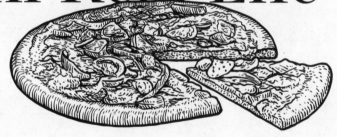

Chapter 12

To Eat Out or Not
to Eat Out?

The people who give you their food give you their heart.
—*Cesar Chavez*

In the rear of a small restaurant abutting the cliffs of Positano, an entire family worked together to prepare and present the diners' orders. There couldn't have been more than three choices of appetizers, five choices of main dishes, and a couple of desserts on offer. Seen through an open door at the back of the establishment, a grandmotherly woman, gray-haired and stooped, carefully tore basil at a well-worn wooden table. Every few minutes she telegraphed a smile to her son, the owner, walking around the dining room, who then would make a stop to chat with a patron. The food was simple and fresh. Its beauty came from the care the family took in preparing the dishes and in highlighting the fresh ingredients grown nearby. There were no tricks of light, no feats of foams. Nothing else needed to be done to the food because it was already perfect.

While such an intimate dining experience in the US is rare, going to restaurants or getting takeout can still be pretty enjoyable. But instead of a special treat, eating out or getting takeout has become commonplace. Most Americans get over one-third of their calories from food prepared outside of their home. This represents double the amount from just a generation earlier despite that eating in restaurants or getting takeout costs more than cooking at home.[207] In addition, when we eat out it is difficult to know what exactly we are consuming.

So if eating at home is cheaper, we are able to prepare a meal in thirty or so minutes, and we have more control over what we are eating, why not do that? Are many of us just lazy and without cooking skills as some have proposed?[208] Maybe, but I think there may be a better explanation. We are busy and overscheduled and overtired. Sometimes we just need help, and that's okay. We can take a break from cooking and still eat food that will nourish us.

When Takeout Is the Only Way Out

Shawn knew that he shouldn't be stopping at the fast-food restaurant after work. He was already taking a medication for his high cholesterol, and I had told him that he might need one for his blood pressure pretty soon. But his last meeting had run over, his wife had picked up their baby and toddler from the daycare after her full day of work, and she had texted him that they were all starving. There weren't enough hours in the day for this harried family during normal times, but now a big project was coming due at work, and Shawn found himself picking up takeout meals at least two times a week. When I asked him about weekends, he looked down at his shoes and decided that, no, it was probably more like three or four times a week, as most of us do.[209] He was just too busy for anything else. He cared about his health but felt as if he already spends his days on a mental treadmill, and if he stopped to change anything, he'd surely fall off and something might break. Shawn knew it would be better and cheaper if he could find the time to cook at home, but he didn't even know where to begin.

Most of my patients, no matter what walk of life they come from, have been a lot like Shawn. They want to make healthy choices, and saving money is always a good idea. The problem is that cooking at home presents several challenges. While we might be able to buy the ingredients needed for a meal and prepare them at home at a fraction of the cost of a restaurant meal, subconsciously we realize there are other hidden costs that encourage us to avoid cooking.

One cost is that fresh, healthy ingredients are prone to spoilage. Something may delay a meal from being made, then when we get around to reaching for the ingredients a day or two later, the meat may have gone off, or veggies have become moldy before we can use them. This waste can quickly discourage the home cook, who now has to carve away large portions of the produce or toss out potentially costly meats and be left with little to make for the dinner they had planned.

An even bigger obstacle to overcome is time. And time isn't free. That doesn't mean we shouldn't cook, only that we need to acknowledge all the costs involved in the process and give a tremendous amount of credit to the people who feed us—effectively sustaining our lives. And if we are the person feeding others, or even just ourselves, we should acknowledge the immense amount of work we are doing. Can we really prepare a meal in thirty minutes or less? Well, it's not so easy. Even if the time listed on the recipe promises a meal in twenty, twenty-five, or thirty minutes, that doesn't account for time needed to meal plan and then drive to the grocery store, shop for the items, drive home, and then put them away—let's break this down and estimate it as adding about ten minutes per dinner per day. If we further consider that the cleanup involved in a home-cooked meal is often fifteen minutes or more, the dinner that our recipe said would take only twenty to twenty-five minutes to prepare is now pushing up against an hour. Excluding potential spoilage, how much additional cost is really involved in home cooking?

According to the Bureau of Labor Statistics, the average hourly wage in 2019 of a worker in the US was around $27.[210] A lot of people make much less, and obviously some make more, but for the sake of this argument that means on average we value fifteen minutes of an American worker's time at around $7. So if a takeout meal for a family of four costs $25 but only requires fifteen minutes to obtain, including picking it up and bringing it to the table, the total cost for that meal is about $32. On the other hand, if ingredients to prepare that meal at home cost a family $15, but the time required to plan, shop for, make, and clean up the meal takes an hour, the meal costs about $42. It isn't really so mysterious to figure out why we eat one-third of our meals out. We aren't lazy or gluttonous. We are tired and are actually being pretty rational consumers about the whole thing.

The problem is that when we eat out or get takeout, it is harder to make good choices. But even if we commit to eating out less, there are going to be days (Friday, I'm looking at you) when we are just too tired or the fridge is too bare to come up with anything reasonable to eat. Even with the best planning, Shawn's family (and possibly yours) is still going to be reliant on picking up dinner once or twice a week. And that's okay. Even if it has to be more than that, it's okay. Mealtime shouldn't be a source of stress.

But when it's time for takeout, it's vital to recognize that there are better options and ways of navigating a menu. Some fast-casual food purveyors have taken the lead in posting their ingredients online, and a few have gone so far as to banish many additives from their menus. To them, on behalf of diet-related disease sufferers everywhere, I want to say thank you. Chipotle says it only uses real ingredients and lists them on its website. The same is true of Sweetgreen, a salad chain that began in Northeastern US cities and is quickly spreading around the country. I could not find any troublesome emulsifiers or additives in its ingredient lists.

Not everyone suffers from diet-related diseases, so it is perhaps a bit self-centered to ask that food purveyors rid their wares of all potential threats to sufferers (who may only represent one in four or five of their customers). But when these restaurants list all of their ingredients for their customers to be able to peruse, we all can make better decisions when going out to eat.

Sadly, many fast-casual food purveyors, even those that purport to be healthy, make finding ingredient lists a challenge, if not impossible. I recently tried to google ingredient lists for dressings at nationally popular salad chains, getting only allergen lists returned for my efforts (save for Sweetgreen). With catchy marketing words such as *natural* and *homemade* on restaurant websites, I knew I was in trouble since these words tell us nothing about what is actually in the products. Because the chains charge a premium for their salads and attempt to cater to a health-conscious group, I thought they might be forthcoming with ingredient lists if I were to contact them. Not so much. Some chains claim that if they were to release ingredient lists, anyone could copy them. As a fan of recipe hacks, I can attest to there being knockoffs of nearly every good dish out there ready to be googled, whether or not ingredient lists are readily available. With the help of industrious cooks posting recipes online, we can make nearly any restaurant dish at home already, but we probably don't for the time-limiting reasons I outlined earlier in this chapter. The restaurants needn't worry!

So why the secrecy around ingredient lists? I believe it is because if we really knew what was going into our food at many of these places, we might not eat it. I don't think the restaurant executives are afraid that home cooks Jim and Joan are going to steal their ideas. Rather, the executives are probably worried that their ingredients will scare Jim and Joan into passing on getting a meal at their establishment.

The Alchemy of Modern Cooking

But it's not just most of the fast-food or fast-casual restaurants that have bombarded their dishes with gut-roiling food additives. Even at high-end restaurants, food additives have not only become accepted, but at many they are embraced as part of the haute cuisine culture. As chefs try to outdo each other with flashier presentations, foams, and air-filled concoctions, they reach for the chemistry that can make it all possible.

The field of molecular gastronomy started to become popular in restaurants in the 1990s. The term *molecular cooking* has been coined to describe using new kitchen equipment resembling a chemistry lab more than your grandmother's stove top, and new ingredients often derived in a laboratory.[211] Some of the best and brightest chefs have become more than amateur chemists, and the most elite culinary schools are teaching molecular gastronomy to their students. A Dublin-based culinary institute gives the following example as a means of instructing students on how they might make an egg-based sauce even creamier:

"The recipe for the egg sabayon included the following ingredients: egg yolk, white refined sugar, water, Irish whiskey, xanthan gum and gellan gum (polysaccharides produced by bacteria), and white coloring. The lightness of the egg-based sauce coupled with the addition of xanthan and gellan gums allowed a stable 'creamlike' layer..."[212]

Molecular gastronomy, invented as a way to create unique treats, has morphed into a cheap shortcut that has now been embraced by food educators and professional chefs alike as not only acceptable, but also capable of elevating food to new heights even while taking our health to new lows. It is now considered food artistry and innovative to add all manner of additives to our foods, in an effort to have the tallest, fluffiest, or most unique preparation of a dish.

In an effort to achieve food artistry, chefs often employ a substance known as agar or agar-agar.[213] It is another long-chain sugar that causes food to gel. Since I usually didn't see this additive listed on ingredient lists, I might not have thought about it if it hadn't made an appearance in the 2021 study that looked at twenty different emulsifiers and their effects on gut bacteria. When it was tested, agar decreased the amounts of what might be considered important anti-inflammatory constituents of our microbiome.[214] And, as with many of the other additives discussed, it is now increasingly available at food markets, especially health food markets, as it is a plant-derived alternative to gelatin.

Ultimately, spending a great deal of money on a meal may have the same effects on our stomach and metabolism as stopping at a drive-through. The effects could be worse since some fast-food purveyors have been making an effort of late to remove food additives. Some restauranteurs are marketing their establishments as healthier, but I retain some skepticism when eating out, regardless of how much money I am spending.

Dining Without Distress

My patients didn't want to isolate themselves, but some have found that to be easier than dealing with the subsequent explosions that followed an evening out. A 2001 study from a family practice journal found "the constant anticipation of the next IBS episode, the need for immediate access to toilet facilities, and the nature of the bowel symptoms often required withdrawal from social activities and resultant isolation."[215] Some formerly gregarious, outgoing people feel like they are being forced to become homebodies. And in the workplace, being seen as antisocial not only impacts one's social life, but it can have career consequences as well.

Eating lunch out with coworkers or when the office orders in is an unavoidable brush with restaurant food. While office group decision-making adds an extra challenge to dining out, and you could always bring a sandwich from home, it is important to figure out how to get along with your friends as well as your bowels.

While eating out will always present more of a challenge than eating at home, I believe that part of the joy of food is enjoying it with friends. There are ways to do so pretty safely. If you've gotten this far, you've read about the common foods sitting on supermarket shelves that can be adulterated. Assume, then, that those same foods or something similar have been purchased by the restaurant kitchen where you are eating. Very few restaurant kitchens make all of their items from scratch, and, as noted earlier, even the more high-end restaurants that do make dishes from scratch may adulterate them on purpose for grander chemistry-driven presentations. The following five simple tips can be used when eating out to help you avoid the additives that may make the next day a lot less fun.

1. **Banish the Bread.** Most restaurants source their bread from commercial bakeries that use the same dough conditioners and stabilizing agents that are in the packages of cheap, shelf-stable white bread at the supermarket. And don't be fooled by the chain sandwich shops that proudly display their breads as freshly baked. They are most likely transported from a massive factory, full of the bad stuff, and just freshly warmed at the store. While you are at it, skip the wraps and tortillas, too. They have the same stuff to promote softness but probably in even greater quantities.

2. **Cancel the Cream.** As noted earlier, cream almost always has food gums or carrageenan in it. Ask about sauces, and if they have cream in them, order something else. Because dairy is often listed as an allergen, servers can find out if a dish has cream in it. Since it is so challenging to get additive-free cream, almost no restaurants in the US have it, and it is safer to assume that a dish with cream is a no-no.

3. **Decline the Dressings.** If you order a salad, ask for some oil and either lemon or balsamic vinegar on the side. Trust no dressing in a restaurant unless you know all the ingredients.

4. **Chuck the Cheese.** Because many restaurants use pre-shredded cheese coated in cellulose, avoid cheeses while eating out unless it is fresh mozzarella, which doesn't have this coating.

5. **Ditch the Dessert.** I hate this one, but desserts usually have many of the additives that have been cited as causing bowel troubles. I know many patients who began to avoid desserts well before

other foods, having first recognized that desserts out were their intestines' downfall.

You may have noticed that the admonishments above sound an awful lot like popular diets such as the Paleo or Whole30 diets. Because these diets are so well known, sometimes the easiest thing to do is tell the waiter you are following one of them. Occasionally a restaurant chain will already have noted which items on their menus are Paleo or Whole30 friendly. Even though you aren't necessarily following these diets, they're shorthand for avoiding foods that probably contain additives, and they are generally understood. Be careful claiming you are gluten-free or dairy-free (unless you are) because many wheat and milk substitutes contain the additives we are trying to avoid in the first place.

Another way to approach eating out is to be sure you are able to identify the ingredients as they appear in their natural state. So instead of mashed potatoes (where adulterated cream or other smoothing ingredients may have been added), order a baked potato with some butter on the side. Instead of ordering chicken slathered in a sauce, order a simple roast chicken breast or quarter that basically still looks like chicken. While there are no guarantees when eating out, choosing food items that are as close as possible to their appearance in nature helps.

Pizza might seem like an impossibility, but there are definitely better choices you can make. While I avoid chains and try to frequent my neighborhood mom-and-pop pizza shop for the simple reason that the food is usually better, another reason is that the mom-and-pops often make their own pizza dough from scratch and from real ingredients. You can ask if they make their own dough and what's in it. Beware the gluten-free doughs (unless you have to avoid gluten for celiac disease) because a gluten-free dough often needs a food gum, most often xanthan gum, to hold it together if the gluten, which is a binder, is missing.

The problem at a lot of pizza places is the cheese, which is often pre-shredded and can contain cellulose and other fillers. Here you have two choices: either get a cheese-less pizza or see if they have fresh mozzarella as an option (sometimes called a margherita pizza on the menu).

Be careful with toppings. Fresh veggies are usually a safe bet, but meats like meatballs, pepperoni, and sausage can contain additives and other ingredients you may want to avoid.

Burgers are a great option when eating out. It's generally the bun you have to worry about. So just skip it. Get a bun-less, cheese-less burger and pile on the veggies instead. Ah, you might be thinking, I can pile on all the lettuce in the world, but burgers still aren't healthy. And perhaps you are right. But I worry less about the meat than the meat substitutes. New nonmeat burgers have been sweeping across restaurants with great fanfare. But these burgers often contain additives like lecithin and cellulose. It's not unreasonable to avoid meat, but please be careful with what you choose to eat instead.

Sandwiches are where things get difficult. This might be American's most popular go-to lunchtime meal, but sandwiches present a really rocky path to navigate. Since this is about eating out, let's assume that packing your own sandwich made of real bread with real cheese and other ingredients is out of the question. Most bread you get from a sandwich shop is not going to be the fresh baked variety made in ovens in the back. Local shops might be a better alternative, but they are often sourcing their bread from nearby commercial bakeries that adulterate their doughs just as the national chains do. Like the Florentine sandwich shop (mentioned in chapter 6) that offered only one kind of bread, sandwich shops offering real bakery breads have limited options, which are likely so delicious you won't want any other kind of bread anyway. But if you can't verify that the bread is without additives, I'd skip the sandwich (or get it without bread, which I guess makes it not a sandwich anymore).

As a final word on the sandwich, be careful of those made with mayonnaise like tuna salad or chicken salad. While some mayos are fine, others have food gums and other additives and are decidedly not. A simple ham and cheese or turkey without cheese, hold the mayo, and then hold the bread may be your best bet.

In general, simple grilled meat, chicken, or fish are probably the best foods to order when faced with a lunchtime challenge. Unless the protein was heavily marinated in a gum- or emulsifier-containing dressing prior to grilling, you should be okay.

Pasta without cheese or cream sauce may be another good go-to. Simple tomato-based sauces are often additive-free. Just remember that meatballs can contain Parmesan cheese coated in cellulose and bread crumbs with all the bread adulterants of sandwiches you are avoiding ordering. A simple pasta and salad with just oil and vinegar is the safest option here.

Tacos and burritos may beat out all of the categories I've just listed. Chipotle has cleaned up its menu, priding itself on offering simple, unadulterated ingredients, and hopefully more chains will follow suit. Until then, going to your neighborhood taco place may be your best bet. If it makes soft tortillas from scratch, consider yourself lucky. If you aren't sure about this, order the hard-shell tacos or dishes without tortillas. Stay away from cheese, sour cream, and guacamole if they aren't freshly made (though the local shops often make them fresh).

Asian takeout places are also great go-tos for healthy (and also not healthy) meals. The variety in just one country is enough to send your head spinning, let alone from the whole continent, so this category is definitely too broad to address in this small amount of space. Briefly, the same rules apply as above; however, a lack of bread and dairy in many cuisines eliminates the need to worry about this step. The big concern here is the sauces. Fish sauce, hoisin sauce, siracha, and others can contain food gums. Try to stay away from the heavily sauced stuff. Stick with steamed dishes or just soy sauce if you can.

Let's Not Forget Breakfast

In my pre-IBS days, breakfast or brunch used to be my favorite meal to eat out. The food could be both a little salty and a little sweet, and the kids weren't cranky yet. It was the perfect time to eat out with delicious food options that were hard to get wrong. But now breakfast can be the most fraught meal to navigate in a restaurant. Unless you are eating at a scratch bakery or a restaurant that sources its breads and pastries from one, these yummy treats are often filled with additives to keep them soft and fresh tasting even when they aren't. Eggs and omelets can contain cream or other non-egg ingredients with their attendant adulterants, and pancakes and waffles may as well. Yogurts, as described previously, aren't always safe. Breakfast sausage can contain basically anything at all.

So what can we do to enjoy eating breakfast out again? Go back to basic principles. Avoid bread and dairy when dining out and order foods that can be closely identified with their original state. A fried egg looks like an egg, breakfast meats that look as close to an intact piece of animal flesh are safest, and don't forget about fruit—it's hard to add anything to plain sliced fruit. Remember to ask if the oatmeal is made with just water and is without other ingredients. If plain oatmeal with a side of fruit doesn't sound like fun restaurant food, well, it's not. Again, a good place to start searching for your additive-free breakfast break is at your locally owned establishments, where they are more likely to be making foods from scratch.

As evidence of how additives can affect our microbiomes continues to emerge, there's hope that not only physicians and dieticians, but also professional chefs and restauranteurs will embrace changing how they prepare food. Until that time comes, we can eat out and try to avoid emulsifiers and thickeners—the more we do it, the more intuitive it becomes.

Chapter 13

How to Eat Everything and Still Lose Weight

and i said to my body. softly. "i want to be your friend."
it took a long breath. and replied,
"i have been waiting my whole life for this."

—*Nayyirah Waheed*

Besides not having to worry about my stomach when I visited Italy, I also didn't have to worry about my waistline, which, at first, I thought was weird. After all, I was eating all of the foods I had been taught would make me gain weight—Roman pasta, Neapolitan pizza, hearty Florentine cuts of meats. I was also eating lots of fresh fruit and vegetables, and I was eating until I was satisfied. When I returned and told friends and colleagues that I had eaten all the sin foods and hadn't gained weight on my trip, many described a similar phenomenon when they had traveled to Italy, Greece, India, and several other countries where fresh whole foods were mainstays of the diet.

It turns out that humans have what weight experts call a set point, or, as some prefer, a settling point. Except for specific periods like growing in childhood, pregnancy, and probably menopause, our bodies aren't necessarily programmed to gain weight (men can also put on weight as they age, but nothing like the sudden change that occurs with pregnancy and menopause). Unfortunately, (for us during modern times, anyway) our bodies may not easily lose the weight, either. Eating real foods in reasonable quantities doesn't usually cause weight gain or, for that matter, weight loss—it doesn't change our settling point. Our bodies, through our fat cells, muscle cells, and microbiome via our brains, tell us how much to eat throughout the day and how much energy to burn. When we eat real food, this system works well and keeps our weight fairly steady.

Eating ultra-processed foods, however, throws this system out of whack, perhaps through chemical signals sent by our microbiome when it digests these substances. While the details are yet to be worked out, what is clear is that eating at least two, but possibly many more, emulsifying and preserving additives causes mice and humans to eat more—a lot more—and causes weight gain—potentially a lot of weight gain.

Does This Microbiome Make Me Look Fat?

We know of thirty hormones and neurotransmitters that affect appetite, the vast majority of which actually tell us to stop eating.[216] While we may be designed to eat, we are also born with over a dozen mechanisms that tell us we've had enough. What's clear is that when we eat ultra-processed foods, that system seems to break down for many of us. While we have to take into account the addictive potential of foods, social cues, and availability, could something else be going on?

Consider the mice introduced in the first chapter that were given the tasteless emulsifiers in their water, gained weight, and developed a condition akin to the metabolic syndrome in humans.[217] The mice consuming the additives had no social pressures on them (as far as I know), were not tasting more sweetness in the food (the food was the same for both groups of mice), and yet the additive-consuming mice were becoming heavier and developing signs of diet-related diseases.

It is well established that some gut bacteria are better than others in extracting the calories from food that the human body doesn't digest on its own. If you have an excess of these bacteria, you will put on more weight eating the same number of calories as a person who has fewer of these bacteria.[218] But you are still deciding how much to eat. A little less established but exciting area of research is trying to answer the question of whether or not the bacteria in our guts can actually override the system and command us to eat more.[219] When our microbiomes digest the food we don't digest, a by-product of their digestion can act as a chemical signaling to our brains. It may be a leap, but it's a short one, to consider that several additives, especially those used in ultra-processed foods, are perhaps encouraging these bacteria to push us to consume more. In any case, something in the ultra-processed food is.

In 2019, scientists housed twenty people in a lab. It was a nice lab, more like a hotel really. Everything they ate was provided to them and recorded. For two weeks they were given a diet of unprocessed foods—no emulsifiers or other additives—just fruit, nuts, veggies, meats, whole grains, and other whole foods. The food looked fairly similar to what I had eaten for much of the time in Italy. Just as I had, the participants could eat as much or as little as they wanted. Then those same people were fed an ultra-processed diet for two weeks with the same additives the mice were given plus a few more—basically stuff that comes wrapped in plastic or is available in the freezer section of the supermarket. Those same people ate an average of 500 calories a day more during the ultra-processed phase of the diet and as a result, they gained about two pounds in two weeks. Everything else during the study was the same—carbs, fats, protein, sleep, exercise, and sodium.

Maybe, you might think, the ultra-processed stuff just tasted better? But no. The scientists running the study accounted for this possibility and also had the participants rate what they thought of the meals. They rated the whole-food diet and the ultra-processed diet similarly. The only difference the study designers allowed for was the food additives and the processing in the ultra-processed foods.[220] And importantly (so I'll say it again), most of these additives aren't food for us—they provide no calories for us—but are a massive food source for our gut bacteria, which may signal us to keep on eating.

We don't eat more food when consuming the natural fibers or prebiotics found in whole foods. So why do we eat more when we consume the prebiotics in the form of emulsifiers and preservatives in ultra-processed food? That isn't clear yet. But eating lots of fresh whole foods on vacation while not eating the ultra-processed stuff is probably why I didn't gain any weight. Still skeptical? Maybe it was all of the walking and sight-seeing I was doing that caused my weight not to budge? That's a reasonable suggestion and one I might have thought, too, before I started caring for patients in the US who move all day long and still struggle with their weight.

Moving More Is Good, But It Isn't Enough

Lena, a thirty-eight-year-old woman, spends her days cleaning houses, working from eight in the morning until three to six in the evening, depending on the day and the number of jobs she has to do. Aside from the time she sits to drive her car from home to home, she spends the rest of her day in constant motion.

While light housekeeping may be what many of us think of when we envision cleaning up, that only approximates what Lena does in the way that a misting rain shower resembles a hurricane. She strips beds, throws laundry in the washer, scrubs bathtubs and showers, and then pushes a heavy vacuum around rooms and up stairs before remaking beds, folding laundry, and heading to her next job. And then she does it again and again before her day is done. Yet Lena struggles with her weight and her blood sugar. She doesn't drink soda very often and doesn't really eat much fast food. But like many of us, Lena eats a lot of ultra-processed breads and other products that throw her ability to self-regulate her weight completely off track. If the key to managing weight is simply moving and avoiding supersize fries, Lena should be fifty pounds lighter with excellent blood sugar. Instead, her numbers are creeping up year after year. It is only after severely restricting ultra-processed foods, and especially ultra-processed carbohydrates, that Lena begins to gain control over her weight and her blood sugar.

If you recall in the introduction the patients on restrictive diets were the ones who clued me in that the type of food wasn't what mattered as much as the avoidance of additives when trying to tame IBS symptoms. So you might be wondering how the diets wound up working for these patients whose primary goal was to lose weight. It turns out that diets can be tricky things. But this isn't news to anyone who has been on a diet before. Some people lose weight, some don't. A few even gain weight on diets that their friends had lost several pounds on. We might be able to blame our microbiomes here, too.

Emerging research suggests that how we process fats, proteins, and carbohydrates not only depends on our own genetic backgrounds, but on the makeup of our microbiomes. Unfortunately, while sometime in the future a lab might be able to analyze your stool and tell you which diet to try first (and, yes, there are labs working on this),[221] right now it's just a matter of trial and error. If you find that you do better avoiding carbohydrates, stick with that. If you do better avoiding fat, then that's a good eating plan for you.

A 2021 study headed by the same lab at the National Institutes of Health that was able to show the weight gain in participants eating ultra-processed food in 2019, looked at whole-food, low-fat diets versus whole-food, low-carbohydrate diets. The study followed the same format that had the participants living at the lab for four weeks, spending two weeks on each diet. No matter which arm of the study they were in, participants lost weight eating a whole-food diet.[222] The key factor that reaches across populations and microbiomes is that if you are able to avoid ultra-processed foods, you are likely to be more successful whichever diet you choose. This assumes you want to lose weight.

By demonizing real food, our diet-obsessed culture has probably made the mess of ultra-processed foods worse, and trying to lose weight or not is a personal choice. Body acceptance is vitally important to our well-being, but it's difficult to achieve. What we should or shouldn't weigh is fraught with stigma, bias, and cultural assumptions. We are all different. If weight loss is not one of your goals, feel free to skip to the next chapter.

Moving Your Settling Point

The good news is the science says you probably won't gain weight if you avoid ultra-processed foods as long as you listen to your body and stop when you are full. The bad news is you probably won't lose weight unless you do a few more things to move your settling point. You do not have to do all five of the things listed. Some of these suggestions just aren't possible for everyone, and that's okay. Do what you can, when you can.

How to move your settling point:

1. Eat real food but not too much (to paraphrase the food writer Michael Pollan)
2. Consider restricting eating by time
3. Exercise to build muscle mass

4. Sleep
5. Reduce stress

Eat Real Food but Not Too Much

We've already reviewed the real food part of this advice. The people who lose weight on restrictive diets do so partly because there are rules around eating—the *not too much* part. But really restrictive rules aren't much fun in the long-term, and few of us can live with them forever (which is why we wind up gaining the weight back). So perhaps we should stop thinking about rules and start thinking about cultural norms.

In some other countries, sweet desserts aren't eaten very often. In others, snacking is extremely uncommon. When I was growing up, my immigrant grandparents had only one large meal midday and had a lighter breakfast and dinner. Our cultural norms today (probably with the help of the ultra-processed food industry) have drifted toward larger portions and lots of snacking. What are some new or, perhaps, old norms that we might incorporate into our lives?

When we give up the ultra-processed foods, it's time to start intuitive eating and paying attention to our hunger cues. Do you normally have a snack before or after lunch? Is it just out of habit, or is it something your body needs? Do you always have dessert after dinner? Again, is this a habit? Perhaps you aren't actually hungry for dessert tonight. Or maybe you are, and skipping dessert is not something you prefer to do. That's okay, too. But we should be intentional about when we eat and how much we eat.

Restrict by Time

If you aren't sure what your body needs due to years of living in a diet-obsessed culture, a popular way to limit eating is to restrict it by time, meaning you can eat what you want but only within certain hours. This is referred to as time-restricted eating, and, as with many guidelines in our diet-crazed culture, it has been taken to an extreme, where some adherents only eat for four hours a day. Besides sounding miserable, that level of restriction isn't sustainable or healthy. Luckily, there is good evidence that fasting for just fourteen hours a day is helpful as part of a comprehensive weight-loss plan. Practically, this may just mean not snacking after dinner.

During a fourteen-hour fast, you can eat for ten hours a day. If you have breakfast at 8 AM, you need to finish dinner by 6 PM. This is potentially difficult with a long work day, so breakfast may need to be later at 9 AM or 10 AM, with dinner finishing at 7 PM or 8 PM. If you find you are hungry and not happy with this, don't do it. If it works for you, great.

There's speculation that time-restricted eating works because the microbiome has something of a diurnal pattern to it, and we shouldn't be feeding it when it should be asleep[223] (also, it is better for weight loss to regularize our sleep patterns). A simpler explanation may be that it keeps us from snacking when we shouldn't be—you won't be able to prop up a bowl of popcorn or chips while watching TV at night. But if you really want that popcorn, go for it. Just ask yourself if you're eating out of habit, because of marketing by the ultra-processed food industry, or because popcorn is something you really enjoy. When we become mindful and intentional about what we are eating, we do much better.

Exercise to Build Muscle

As we age, we lose muscle mass. The amount of fat in our bodies increases as our muscle mass decreases. This is bad for weight regulation because both fat and muscle make hormones that tell us whether to eat or not to eat. Perhaps this developed through evolution because when our ancestors worked hard, it wasn't to their advantage to want to eat all the time. On the other hand, when they were sedentary and storing fat, their bodies may have learned to keep packing on the pounds during a period of relative calm. In any case, having more fat cells works to our disadvantage, and having more muscle works to our advantage from a weight-loss perspective.

Aerobic exercise, like fast walking, running, cycling, and playing sports, is great for many reasons, but it may not cause a whole lot of weight loss[224] (though it can definitely help maintain weight). Aerobic exercises are good for cardiovascular fitness, and you should do them, but building muscle is important for weight loss.

There are plenty of books and personal training videos that can help you build muscle through isotonic exercise like weight lifting or isometric exercise like yoga or Pilates. Find what you like doing to keep moving, but don't leave out the muscle-building part. You don't need to become a professional weight lifter, but as you age, you need to at least maintain what you had in your twenties or, in many cases, try to reclaim it.

Sleep

As already mentioned, regular sleep helps maintain weight. Night shift work, switching sleeping patterns between days and nights, or just not getting enough sleep contributes to weight gain and makes it relatively more difficult to lose weight. Telling a night shift worker not to work nights is pretty silly. Working nights, at least for hospital employees, is often better paying. Night shift work is routinely assigned to new doctors and nurses, police officers, and other essential workers. It isn't a choice for them. It is an obstacle for weight loss, but if the first three suggestions are followed, it can be overcome. Those who can go to bed at a reasonable hour, should do so. Your body will thank you. If you have trouble with insomnia, consider cognitive behavioral therapy for insomnia that your health care professional might be able to tell you more about. I do not advocate using pharmacologic sleep aids with rare exceptions because many of them have been associated with weight gain, among other problematic side effects.

Reduce Stress

Having more stress certainly contributes to weight gain. I have generally found that people who have a great deal of stress already know they have a great deal of stress. Pointing that out and telling them to relax or de-stress isn't terribly helpful. Most likely they've heard of meditation and exercise as de-stressing methods. They'd love to take a vacation to the South of France or Hawaii. Odds are pretty good that whatever is causing their stress is also prohibiting them from doing the things that would reduce their stress. If they had more money, they could go on a great trip to de-stress, but if they had the money, they might not be so stressed in the first place. If they had more time to meditate, they might not be so stressed, but then if they had that time, they also wouldn't be so stressed. Telling a person with a stressful life to just have less stress is like telling a person with depression to just be less sad—it's not terribly constructive advice. That doesn't mean stress reduction can't be worked on, just that it is potentially much harder to do than any of the other steps above. I would urge you to consider what brings you peace and joy and, if you are able, to find some moments for them. Stress reduction can have far-reaching effects on our bodies.

Having said that, if any of the steps above are too difficult to do at the moment, don't worry about it. My patients have taught me that the main problem causing our weight gain isn't lack of movement or lack of sleep or even too much stress (although these things are contributors). It is what we are eating. Get rid of the ultra-processed stuff, eat everything real, and still lose or maintain your weight.

Chapter 14

Troubleshooting

When you have eliminated the impossible, whatever remains, however improbable, must be the truth.

—*Sir Arthur Conan Doyle*

When I was beginning my training as an internist, a thirty-five-year-old woman came into the clinic. Charlotte felt miserable—her periods were unbearably heavy, she was anemic, she seemed to be putting on weight, and she was tired all the time. After a brief workup, it was clear what Charlotte's problem was, or at least I thought it was. Her labs came back showing significant hypothyroidism—meaning her thyroid gland was unable to produce enough thyroid hormone for her body to properly regulate her periods or her weight. I thought the anemia and fatigue were also related. There was an easy fix—I prescribed thyroid hormone for Charlotte and saw her back six weeks later, expecting to have solved her problem. But Charlotte was no better. If anything, she felt worse. Her TSH, a measure of how well the level of thyroid hormone I had prescribed was meeting her needs, was not much better than it had been before she began taking the medication. I increased her dose and told her to come back in six weeks. Six weeks later, Charlotte's TSH was even worse. I went to a senior physician and asked what I should do.

"That's a high enough dose for a woman of her size even if her own thyroid isn't making any hormone at all," he told me. "She must not be taking it."

"But she is," I insisted.

Charlotte was a working mother with two kids. She didn't have time to be tired or anemic or have heavy periods.

"Secondary gain," the senior physician shrugged. "Find out why she's not taking the medication."

By *secondary gain*, he was implying that Charlotte was getting something out of feeling unwell—sympathy or support or any number of things. That she wasn't getting better must be her fault since we had done everything right.

Or had we? No, I thought. There's something else going on. I went back to talk to Charlotte.

"What are your bowels like?" I asked her.

"What they've always been like," she told me. "I can go once a day, or not for two days, or three times in a day. That's just me."

"Do you ever have diarrhea?" I asked.

"Sometimes," she sighed, seemingly resigned to it. "I've been like this for years. They told me I had IBS when I was around twenty."

"I want to do a blood test for something called celiac disease," I told her. "I don't think you're absorbing your thyroid medication, and I want to find out why."

A week later, I called Charlotte. She had tested as having celiac disease. I referred her to a gastroenterologist and a biopsy proved that she did indeed have celiac. Problem solved. I felt great. Unfortunately, Charlotte felt no better. Her thyroid still wasn't right, and despite getting rid of all the gluten in her diet (something sufferers of celiac disease must do), Charlotte was no better. Over the next several months, she kept her food separate from that of the rest of the family and bought kitchen utensils that were only used for her food. I couldn't figure out why Charlotte wasn't getting any better.

And then one day her gastroenterologist called me.

She learned that Charlotte had a weekend job as a server in a pizzeria and thought the airborne flour from the dough that was being made in the kitchen was getting into her system. And she was right. Charlotte was able to quit her part-time job at the pizzeria, and her celiac tests returned to normal, her thyroid was regulated, and she finally felt great.

I was fortunate to have met Charlotte so early in my career because she taught me that if a patient isn't getting better, to keep looking for something else. And then if she still isn't getting better, look again. And if that doesn't work, make sure that you call for help—someone else may have a better idea. There is a reason a patient isn't getting better—that they aren't trying hard enough isn't likely to be it.

So if you aren't getting better after removing the additives mentioned in this book, it isn't your fault. But it is important to try to figure out what else might be going on.

Getting the Right Diagnosis

No one should be using this book to get a diagnosis. If you have bowel troubles or other health ailments, you should be under the care of a doctor. Getting rid of emulsifiers and other additives is a strong foundation on which to build good health, but it isn't the answer to everything that ails us. Our bodies are complicated and constantly changing. Sometimes there is a simple solution, and sometimes there isn't. If you're not feeling right, it is vital that you get the answers as to why.

As mentioned several times in this book, your microbiome can turn over fast. If you haven't noticed a difference after a week of eliminating emulsifiers and trying to eat a whole-food diet, it's time to start troubleshooting. First, keep a three-day journal of everything that goes in your mouth—even if it is just a sip of something or a piece of gum or a vitamin—write it down. When you have some time, make sure you check the ingredients of everything you've written down. If you haven't been eating out and know everything you have been eating and still don't feel right, it's time to consult with a health care professional.

Charlotte had both a thyroid problem and celiac disease. She never had IBS. She was misdiagnosed and then undiagnosed for too long. But when Charlotte was told she had IBS in the 1980s, there wasn't a great blood test for celiac disease—the test I was able to do came along in the early 2000s.

You may have been carrying a diagnosis for a long time, and it may be right. But if you don't feel better, consider that it might not be and see your doctor for more help.

Repopulating Your Microbiome

You've been to your doctor and are positive that you have the right diagnosis or at least are on the right track. You've done your food journaling and are sure that you are avoiding all the emulsifiers and thickeners mentioned in this book. And maybe things still aren't right. As mentioned previously, so much rests on your microbiome, and the more ultra-processed foods you've consumed in your lifetime, the fewer good bacteria you have to work with.[225]

As dietician and University of Massachusetts professor Barbara Olendzki told me, it is important to get rid of the microbiome-changing additives, but it is also important to build up a good microbiome with proper nutrition. So where can we find these good bacteria?

Although I wish for a time when we can go to the store and pick up some microbiome-building pills, that time isn't right now. Probiotics in a pill may be of questionable value (see "The Probiotic Problem" in chapter 3). Some people will swear by them, but there just isn't enough evidence for me to recommend one over another. Like so much in the unregulated supplement industry, it is extremely difficult to know what you are really getting.

Thanks to research done on fermented foods, we do know where we can find probiotics and how to possibly make them flourish in our own guts—probiotics are hanging out in most grocery refrigerators. Real yogurt and kefir (yogurt drink) are great probiotic options if you are a dairy eater. If you aren't a dairy eater, look for coconut-based alternatives with live cultures, since coconut milk can be creamy on its own without additives (the others tend to need thickeners to create something resembling yogurt). Kimchi and sauerkraut are for cabbage lovers. If you don't like dairy or cabbage, it may be worth giving kombucha a try—it's like a fizzy flavored tea. Although it can be pricey, it isn't terribly hard to make. These, along with other fermented foods, can introduce new and hopefully beneficial bacteria to your gut as demonstrated in the Stanford study that showed increasing gut diversity and decreasing markers of inflammation in people who consumed them.[226]

Just as any living creatures need to be fed regularly if they are going to survive, introducing new gut flora and then leaving them to starve won't be helpful in the long-term. You have to fertilize your lovely garden with whole grains, fruits, and vegetables. But what if you don't like fermented foods? Is there any other way to repopulate your microbiomes?

We've already established that good bacteria and fungi are in our guts. It turns out bacteria and fungi are everywhere. And lots of them are in actual gardens. Although there is currently scant research on gardening to improve our microbiomes, it makes sense that contact with the outdoors would increase the diversity of our own little ecosystems.[227] To test this hypothesis, researchers conducted a small study comparing the microbiomes of gardening families to non-gardening families and did find a difference.[228] Will gardening pan out as a way to improve our gut microbiomes? Maybe. In the meantime, it's a great way to get the kids out of the house, get some exercise, and grow tasty food. If it improves your gut, all the better.

Is there a way to feed the good bacteria in our guts while starving the bad? I would propose that there is and that our ancestors figured it out for us by deciding what we should and shouldn't eat. This doesn't mean we all need to be Paleo adherents. In this case, eating everything means eating everything our ancestors did before indoor plumbing—bowel troubles caused by dietary missteps would have been a much bigger deal before toilet paper and flush toilets. We became symbiotic with our microbiomes through the food we ate. We kept the good stuff growing in our guts and were rewarded with excellent bowel health as payment for our efforts.

Hope for the Future?

Researchers across the world are trying to figure out what an ideal microbiome might look like, in whom, and how we might nurture our personal microbiome. In Israel, Dr. Eran Elinav's laboratory is trying to sort out which diet might work best, depending on what an individual's microbiome looks like.[229] In the UK in collaboration with American scientists, Dr. Timothy Spector's PREDICT studies are attempting something similar while also tracking blood sugar, cholesterol, and other lab values. According to the PREDICT 2 study summary, "the best diet to prevent disease needs matching to a person's gut microbiome and it might be possible to find personalised foods or diets that will help reduce the chance of developing chronic disease as well as metabolic syndrome."[230]

So perhaps one day not too far off in the future, we will learn exactly which foods our most beneficial gut residents prefer instead of having to make broadly applicable guesses. And maybe in repayment for our nourishing them even better, we will be rewarded with ever-improving health.

Meanwhile, other scientists are hard at work to sort out how to deliver better bacteria and fungi to our guts. It has long been known that doing a fecal transplant—infusing the colon with someone else's stool—could treat a sometimes life-threatening infection called *Clostridium difficile*, or *c. diff*. Some treated patients had been observed to have improvements in other conditions as well, so a 2019 study infused the colons of patients suffering with IBS with stool from a super-pooper donor. It is unclear how the thirty-six-year-old male donor was recruited for this particular honor, but his stool was used in over one hundred IBS patients. Fifty-five were given approximately a toothpaste tube's worth of his stool, and the same number were given half that amount. Another group received their own stool as a placebo.[231] Almost all of the patients who received the larger dose of stool improved as far out as three months post–fecal transplantation. More than three-quarters improved with the smaller dose. The microbiomes of the groups that received the fecal transplants changed, becoming more like that of the donor stool.

But super poop is not a cure-all. Stool carries disease. With the regulatory environment getting more challenging, one of the more ambitious projects, started at the Massachusetts Institute of Technology to supply donor poop to all who might need it, recently began the process of shutting down. In its place, for better (definitely cleaner) or for worse (these are likely to be pricey), private companies are trying to develop super-poop bacteria in a pill that will survive on their way to our intestines. But in their quest to clean up the disease-causing bacteria, these poop pills may not be as effective as the whole stool.[232] So we are stuck waiting for this technology to catch up, too.

Persistently High Blood Sugars and Other Lab Abnormalities

If you've tried to eliminate the additives mentioned in this book, cut down on your ultra-processed food intake, and still have lab abnormalities, it's time to see your doctor again (because your doctor should have been involved already if you've had abnormal blood work). If you've been suffering with high blood sugars for a while, your pancreas may not have enough reserve to manage even fewer carbohydrates. Since diabetes is a progressive disease, it does become more difficult over time to manage, and diet alone may no longer be able to combat high blood sugars. Even diet combined with one or two medications may not be enough. I advise my patients with diabetes to cut down on their carbohydrate intake to 150, sometimes 100, grams a day. If you want to cut down even more, it is best to consult with a dietician and your physician because things can start to get trickier and closer monitoring is warranted.

If your cholesterol is still elevated, medication or a medication adjustment, if you are already taking medication, may be needed. For those with familial syndromes, diet just isn't enough. Sometimes genetics makes it difficult to get cholesterol in a good range even when eating a strictly whole-food diet.

Never ignore abnormal liver tests or significantly elevated inflammatory markers. If they remain elevated despite best dietary efforts, please make sure that you have had a thorough workup and you know why they are elevated.

Staying Regular

With the exception of traditional societies near the arctic circle, where vegetation struggles to grow for much of the year, it should be noted that the vast majority of traditional diets are firmly rooted in plants. Our bowels generally feel much better when provided with lots of fruits and veggies. I'm not going to tell you how much of them to eat. What I will say is that there are some general principles applicable to most people regarding eating plant-based items to regulate their bowels.

If you have kids, you have probably been given this advice by your pediatrician at some point. As discussed previously, most adults have boundaries when it comes to discussing their bowels. Not only do children have no boundaries when it comes to waxing poetic about their poop, but when they have a problem, it quickly becomes their parents' problem, too. The parents promptly call the pediatrician for their kids, whereas they may not call their own doctors when experiencing similar difficulties. Suffice it to say that pediatricians deal with a lot of bowel issues. So I've borrowed heavily from my pediatrician colleagues here.

The best piece of advice I've heard from pediatricians to help regulate constipated bowels is to eat two fruits beginning with the letter *p* every day. (The *p* also stands for poop! Pediatricians are fun like that.) So peaches, plums, pineapples, papayas, prunes (you knew that one), and pears. It works for adults, too. The reason these fruits are so popular with kids is that they are sweet. If you want some less sweet bowel movers, then the old standbys of beans, oatmeal, and other whole grains are a great grown-up go-to, in order to be able to go. A hearty tablespoon or two of chia seeds mixed into yogurt or made into a chia pudding with milk or your favorite gum-free milk substitute, are other great ways to stay regular.

For problems with looser stools or diarrhea, my pediatrician friends recommend the BRAT diet (bananas, rice, and toast). Basically, these foods will bind you up. If you are having trouble with constipation, however, bananas, rice, and breads should be avoided.

Areas of the world where people consume a lot of bread—Italy for example—also consume a lot of vegetables and fruit. In India, rice and naan are often accompanied by dishes heavy in veggies and lentils. In Latin America, rice is often served with beans. There is a balance in traditional dishes of foods that move the bowels along with foods that don't. If you are getting constipated after getting rid of all the emulsifiers and other additives that speed things up, consider that you may be eating too heavily from the constipating groups and try to balance meals by reaching for more movers. Remember that what you feed yourself, you are also feeding your microbiome.

Poop Is Still Too Loose

Sometimes the cause of loose stools isn't a mystery, but it can be surprising. I remember a perfectly healthy young patient who tested as having *c. diff* without the usual risk factors of having taken antibiotics or being immunosuppressed. That she worked in a hospital was the only way we could figure she picked up the problematic bug—although she always wore the proper protection when seeing patients with *c. diff.* Another patient, a healthy suburban mom who didn't like camping and wouldn't even know where to find a water well wound up with giardia—an intestinal parasite found in untreated water supplies. We considered that it may have come from her dog, a fairly uncommon route of transmission. Both of these patients had minor symptoms of these intestinal invaders, though other patients can get so sick as to require hospitalization with these bugs. Unfortunately, no amount of whole foods was going to help. They needed antibiotics. Sometimes we can't fight the nasty bacteria that have set up shop in our guts without some help, and that's okay. And sometimes, unfortunately, the pills we take to help our bodies recover wind up causing looser stools.

Metformin, taken for elevated blood sugars, is probably one of the biggest offenders here. But it is a great medication for a lot of people with diabetes and can also help with a few other diagnoses. It is important to start with a low dose of this medication and to always take it with food to help reduce stomach upset. Besides metformin, antidepressants, high blood pressure medications, and medications that reduce stomach acid commonly can loosen stools. If you are on these medications and think they may be causing diarrhea, do not stop taking them, but do talk with your doctor about possible alternatives.

In the meantime, if your stools are loose, consider eating more foods that can bind things up and slow things down as noted above. And be careful of juices and large fructose loads because they can overwhelm your gut.

Poop Is Still Too Hard

If you've removed emulsifiers from your diet and have increased your whole-food consumption but are still constipated, you can try a few tricks to get things moving. Make sure you are drinking enough water. If you aren't drinking enough, your body will conserve water where it can, and your stool will get hard as your body uses the water that your colon normally would for more important functions. How much is enough? You don't need your urine to be clear, but if you find that your urine is consistently dark yellow, you probably need to drink more. If you haven't been exercising much, know that the more you move, the more your bowels are likely to move. Besides that, consider the *p* fruits and avoid the constipating foods as noted above.

You can also consider coffee—another real-food mover and a little bit of a mystery. In studies, both caffeinated and decaffeinated coffee helped people poop, so it's not the caffeine. Warm water didn't have the same effect, so temperature isn't the driver, either.[233] Coffee has hundreds of compounds possibly working together to stimulate our intestines to get moving. We may not know why for a while, but coffee is another great example of a whole food working its magic.

If you are still having trouble getting things moving, review your medication list with your doctor. The list of medications that can induce constipation is long and includes pain medication, blood pressure medication, and antidepressants. Other medication options may work for you that are less constipation inducing.

Also make sure to review your supplement list. Iron and calcium can slow down the bowels tremendously. Ask your doctor if getting these minerals from real food might be a better choice for you. Or perhaps inquire whether a magnesium supplement might help. Magnesium has been a game-changer for many of my patients, though the pill form can be hit or miss. I often recommend a powder that can be mixed with water (but avoid the flavored ones if they have the additives we have discussed). Start with a small amount and increase slowly because magnesium can really get things going.

Diarrhea or Constipation, Depending on the Time of Month

If you happen to possess ovaries, perhaps you've noticed a particular pattern to your stubborn bowels. In 2014, a group of researchers decided to query women about gastrointestinal symptoms when they came in to see their gynecologist for a routine exam. They had no medical diagnoses and weren't coming in to discuss their intestinal health, and yet, when queried, a quarter of them reported diarrhea just before and during their periods.[234] Let me be clear that these participants did not suffer from IBS or any other diagnosis. This was their normal pattern, but these symptoms can be much more difficult in people already struggling with bowel ailments. In another study, patients with intestinal disease diagnoses experienced rates of alternating constipation and diarrhea with their menstrual cycles at twice the rate of people without such diagnoses.[235]

For years, women have been telling me that around the time of ovulation they experience symptoms of constipation (ovulation occurs about two weeks after the first day of your last period), and right before and during menstruation they get more gas, looser stools, or diarrhea. Why does this happen?

Well, around the time of one's period, levels of prostaglandins increase. Prostaglandins help bowels get a little looser in the body. In susceptible people, a surge of prostaglandins can cause the colon to empty its contents fairly quickly. Around ovulation time, levels of progesterone increase dramatically. Progesterone can cause the gastrointestinal tract to slow down.[236] It may also contribute to why some women become constipated during pregnancy.[237] But unfortunately, this is poorly understood. Women's health, in general, is a subject in need of much more study.

For now, knowing what to expect can be a big help. If you've found that you experience more constipation a week or so after your period ends, that's the time to heed the advice for constipated patients in the section above. If your period is regular, you might even be able to head things off by eating lots of vegetables, fruits, and whole grains in the days preceding ovulation. Then when bowels start to get a little looser, or if you are able to predict when your period will come, try eating more constipating foods like rice and bananas just before and during your period. It might not be a perfect solution, but it should help.

You can use a period tracker app if you aren't sure whether your cycle might be contributing to your bowel symptoms. It's also probably worth talking to your primary care or women's health professional about your symptoms. Medications can help regulate your cycle or ease symptoms if changing your diet isn't doing enough.

The important thing is that if your body is giving you trouble, don't give up. There are many possible reasons you may not feel well. Make sure you have a health care team that keeps looking for answers and solutions that work for you.

Conclusion

Cooking Up Change

Food is everything we are. It's an extension of nationalist feeling, ethnic feeling, your personal history, your province, your region, your tribe, your grandma. It's inseparable from those from the get-go.

—*Anthony Bourdain*

In light of what we've learned this past decade, it's time to take a step back and reconsider how we look at food and examine how the foods we eat interact with our bodies and our microbiomes. It is going to require a whole new way of thinking about additives—not assuming they are safe based on their original food sources or that they are safe for long-term consumption based on studies in healthy individuals that may have only lasted a few days.

A universal movement away from additives would completely upend the way we think about food and rock the very foundation upon which the entire food industry has been built. Dr. Monteiro at the University of São Paulo calls this a David versus Goliath problem, with the inadequately funded scientists and public health leaders trying to battle a multitrillion-dollar, global ultra-processed food behemoth.[238] We need to re-evaluate the safety of food additives in light of the new evidence that some of them are likely contributing to the rise of a variety of diseases. The prevailing nutrition paradigm—how we think about food— had not considered whole foods, additives, or the microbiome very much in the past, although it is now becoming increasingly recognized as vitally important to human health.

179

Still, I believe the emerging science on the microbiome and food has the potential to be revolutionary. Antibiotics revolutionized modern medicine. Having the ability to conquer strep throat, for instance, has rendered a common childhood illness that once caused devastating heart disease into a nuisance. Being able to treat bacterial skin infections that just a few generations ago resulted in amputations has allowed us to become more cavalier about cuts and abrasions. Discovering how to kill disease-causing bacteria has greatly improved the health of billions around the world. It isn't that far-fetched to imagine that learning how to cultivate the good microorganisms to our advantage might have similarly wide-ranging health impacts.

Unfortunately, unlike with these earlier breakthroughs, there isn't going to be a simple pill we can take—at least not for a while. It is going to take a shift in how we do things, and that's a bit harder, made even more challenging by those who are profiting off our eating habits. Dr. Monteiro explained:

> Paradigms, we know that they take some time to change, but the speed [of this change] is really very slow. What explains that is the profits— the political economy of the ultra-processed foods. These companies are so powerful, they are able to prolong the time needed to shift the paradigm . . . What can be a game-changer is the evidence that these products can really harm health in very important ways. When it was clear that tobacco was decreasing productivity of workers and increasing the cost of health services, it was clear that tobacco was bad for the whole economy. It was only good for the tobacco industry. I think one day we will arrive in a [similar] situation [with ultra-processed foods]. The rest of the [world] will say, "No, this is not good. There are some companies that are profiting from this, but it is very bad for the rest of society."

It is becoming increasingly clear that many disease sufferers seem to do a lot better when not ingesting emulsifiers and other gut microbiome-altering additives. Recently begun studies in the UK, FADiets and the Mechanistic Nutrition in Health (MECNUT) Emulsifier project, hope to find out if certain emulsifiers might cause problems in human beings. But the results of these studies will take years. Moreover, they are being done in small groups of volunteers who may not suffer from all of the conditions that we are concerned with.

A much larger trial being done in France called the NutriNet-Santé study is looking more broadly at the effects of ultra-processed foods on disease across a wide swath of the population. This study is already finding evidence that consuming more ultra-processed foods leads to appreciably higher rates of disease but is not set up to identify the components of the ultra-processed foods that are responsible. So additive-specific and disease-specific answers may be even further away. In the meantime, the available evidence is strong enough for France and Brazil to have issued guidelines to their populations recommending they avoid additive-laden foods.[239]

Dr. Chassaing has a cross-Atlantic perspective, having done his postdoctoral studies and becoming an assistant professor at Georgia State University before returning to his native France in 2018. He told me, as Dr. Monteiro mentioned of Brazilians, that French people are becoming more aware of the damage food additives can do, and that additive-free foods are a trend in France that he hopes will become increasingly popular as the evidence for avoiding them builds. He asked me if we might have something similar going on in the US these days. I had to admit we do not. We have supermarket shelves lined with products that often contain additives but claim to be gluten-free or preservative-free or even all-natural because technically the additives were extracted from natural sources.

Sometimes I like to dream of a world where an adulterated food needs to be clearly marked as such. But that's not the reality right now. I have yet to find reliable wording on packaging in the US that indicates the product is free of emulsifiers and other nonfood additives.

We may have to do a little more work in countries where additive-free foods have yet to catch on, and the burden of making our food more microbiome-friendly will have to rest with consumers for the time being. But this is not at all an impossible task, whether or not we have regulations or our food is labeled as "additive-free." As Dr. Monteiro explained, we don't need to eat ultra-processed foods at all.

The more we become aware of what we are putting into our bodies and demand change, the more likely we are to get it. Knowledge is power, but so is money. It is recommended that a family of four budget $1,000 a month for food.[240] That's a lot of money to use to demand change. People are already spending their money on healthier foods, encouraging better options from those who supply our food. More quick-serve restaurants are offering whole food–based options, and traditional fast-food chains are picking up on the trend as well.[241] Whether at a restaurant or at home, eating should be joyful and full of healthy choices. If we can vote with our dollars by choosing additive-free, emulsifier-free, and microbiome-friendly foods more often, then the industry will take note. Working toward good health is a journey, but there's no reason it shouldn't be a delicious one.

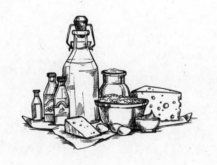

Appendix A

Additives to Avoid (and Why)

The following lists are sorted by chemical category and provide more information on the additives to avoid that were addressed throughout *Eat Everything*. It was generated by considering which ingredients seem to be ubiquitous in ultra-processed foods in the US and then looking at the data behind these additives to assess which have been shown to have gastrointestinal and metabolic side effects. If an additive did not have data suggesting gastrointestinal or metabolic side effects, it was not included. That doesn't mean that all other additives are good for you, but we have to start somewhere, and we have to exist in an imperfect world.

This was not a scientific study but rather a combination of evidence from several different studies. I mainly relied on existing studies and patient self-reports of the additives that seemed to most upset their systems. While I wish there was more evidence on specific additives in specific patient populations, the evidence building against these additives is generally much more robust than the evidence that got them approved in the first place. If the small studies that resulted in approval were enough to put them into your food, I figure that small studies raising safety questions should be enough to take them out for a few weeks and see how much better you do.

Top Twenty-Four Additives to Avoid, Listed Alphabetically

Acacia Gum	Maltodextrin
Agar-Agar	Mannitol
Carob Bean Gum	Modified (fill-in-the-blank)
Carrageenan	Starch
Cellulose	Mono- and diglycerides
Cellulose Gum	Polysorbate 60 and 80
(Carboxymethylcellulose)	Sorbitol
High-Fructose Corn Syrup	Soy and Sunflower Lecithin
Gellan Gum	Stevia
Glycerol	Sucralose
Guar Gum	Titanium Dioxide
Inulin (Chicory Root Extract)	Xanthan Gum
Locust Bean Gum	Xylitol
(Carob Bean Gum)	

I gave up these ingredients myself (not terribly hard because the types of foods that have one, often have several additives) and then encouraged patients like the ones I discussed in the book to do something similar. I still eat some of the items, like high-fructose corn syrup, in small quantities. This is not only because it is so hard to avoid them completely, but also because the science I've read says that in small quantities, they are likely to be digested just fine. I've completely sworn off others, like food gums, carrageenan, and maltodextrin, and suggest that my patients do the same.

These aren't all the food additives out there. And these aren't all of the items that you may need to avoid for all of your particular health reasons. I encourage anyone with health ailments to discuss what they eat with their doctors.

Nothing is all good or all bad, and if an additive has been noted to do something good, I mention that as well. But on balance, I believe the evidence points to the bad outweighing the good for these additives for sufferers of diet-related diseases. Without a doubt, new additives will already have been introduced since the writing of this book. The key to managing the deluge of additives is to remember to stick to whole foods as much as possible. Since additives can be studied for decades and still be controversial, there will always be disagreement. However, in the past several years, sticking as much as possible to whole foods has been an unusual point of agreement among cardiologists[242] and gastroenterologists,[243] and has been included in the national guidelines of countries such as Brazil[244] and Uruguay,[245] with many others likely to follow suit.

Cultures have known about the benefits of eating whole foods for a long time. I've learned from the Italians to keep food simple. If there is something your food doesn't need, leave it out. The bottom line is you don't need any of these additives, and there is no compelling reason for them to be in your food. Avoid them for at least a week and then see if you are spending less time thinking about your gut and more time feeling much better.

Simple Sugars and Sweeteners

A simple sugar is a carbohydrate that is generally chemically simple, with fewer atoms and bonds than other carbohydrates, but not all of them can be broken down so easily by our gastrointestinal systems. The ones listed below need some help or are nondigestible (hence, the lack of calories in sweeteners that aren't sugar).

High-fructose corn syrup (HFCS)
Can the human body digest this? Not well in large doses
Do some gut bacteria digest this? Yes
Can it alter the gut microbiome? Possibly[246]
Can it cause inflammation? Yes (perhaps inducing NAFLD)
Possible immediate effects of consuming HFCS: Diarrhea,
    bloating, gas. These effects might be exacerbated when
    consumed with modified food starches as shown in a study
    of toddlers with diarrhea.[247]
Possible long-term effects of consuming HFCS: Diabetes,[248]
    elevated triglycerides/cholesterol,[249] fatty liver disease,[250]
    colon cancer[251]

Stevia (Stevioside)—*technically a glycoside (a simple sugar with a few extra atoms) but classified here as a simple sugar so we don't get too complicated*

Can the human body digest this? No

Do some gut bacteria digest this? Yes[252]

Can it alter the gut microbiome? Probably

Possible immediate effects of consuming Stevia: Diarrhea and bloating[253] (if erythritol, a polyol, like xylitol, listed below, has been added—which it often has been)

Possible long-term effects of consuming Stevia: Unknown

Sucralose

Can the human body digest this? No

Do some gut bacteria digest this? A little

Can it alter the gut microbiome? Yes[254]

Can it cause inflammation? Maybe[255]

Possible immediate effects of consuming sucralose: Diarrhea, bloating, gas

Possible long-term effects of consuming sucralose: Unknown

Complex Sugars, Gums, and Starches

This is where the terminology can get a little confusing. Polysaccharides are complex sugars—sometimes containing way more molecules than simple sugars—and are often more challenging to break down. Different components of the microbiome prefer different "foods," and even though they are lumped together, it is likely that the effects of each of these substances vary greatly.

Polysaccharides include starches, which are basically long chains of glucose sugar; and fibers, which can be almost anything else. The fibers are further classified, but those categories, like soluble and insoluble fiber, were set up based on how the substances reacted in the lab and actually tell us very little about what our microbiomes do with them.[256] Some polysaccharides, like cellulose, make up the cell walls of plants and can be beneficial when in their whole-food form.

When they are removed from the plant and used as an additive, they may be broken down earlier in the digestive tract and may be more easily consumed by not-so-friendly bacteria.[257]

Food gums are technically a type of fiber and can vary quite a bit from one another. Are some better than others? Probably. Do we have enough data yet to know which are? We do not. Fiber is still something of a black box—we don't have clear-cut science on how different processing (and ultra-processing) leads to changes in digestion and the microbiome.[258] Bottom line? Stick with whole foods as much as possible and avoid the following fiber additives.

Agar-Agar
Can the human body digest this? Yes
Do some gut bacteria digest this? Yes
Can it alter the gut microbiome? Maybe[259]
Can it cause inflammation? Unknown
Possible immediate effects of consuming agar-agar: Diarrhea, bloating
Possible long-term effects of consuming agar-agar: Unknown

Carrageenan
Can the human body digest this? No
Do some gut bacteria digest this? Yes
Can it alter the gut microbiome? Yes[260]
Can it cause inflammation? Yes[261]
Possible immediate effects of consuming carrageenan: Abdominal pain and diarrhea
Possible long-term effects of consuming carrageenan: Crohn's disease or UC in genetically or microbiome-susceptible individuals[262]

Cellulose—*only avoid when listed as an additive—it also makes up the cell walls of actual plants, and is beneficial in the form of fruits and vegetables*
Can the human body digest this? No

Do some gut bacteria digest this? Yes, depending on the
microbiome[263]

Can it alter the gut microbiome? Yes[264]

Can it cause inflammation? Probably not

Possible immediate effects of consuming cellulose: Diarrhea,
bloating, gas

Possible long-term effects of consuming cellulose: Probably none

Acacia Gum (Gum Arabic)

Can the human body digest this? No

Do some gut bacteria digest this? Yes

Can it alter the gut microbiome? Yes[265]

Can it cause inflammation? Probably not

Possible immediate effects of consuming acacia gum: Diarrhea,
bloating, gas[266]

Possible long-term effects of consuming acacia gum: Probably
none

Cellulose Gum (Carboxymethylcellulose)

Can the human body digest this? No

Do some gut bacteria digest this? Yes

Can it alter the gut microbiome? Yes

Possible immediate effects of consuming cellulose gum: Diarrhea,
bloating, gas[267]

Possible long-term effects of consuming cellulose gum: Intestinal
ulceration and inflammation (IBD) in genetically susceptible
individuals[268]

Gellan Gum

Can the human body digest this? No

Do some gut bacteria digest this? Yes

Can it alter the gut microbiome? Probably

Can it cause inflammation? Probably not

Possible immediate effects of consuming gellan gum: Diarrhea[269]
Possible long-term effects of consuming gellan gum: Unknown

Guar Gum
Can the human body digest this? No
Do some gut bacteria digest this? Yes
Can it alter the gut microbiome? Yes
Can it cause inflammation? Probably not
Possible immediate effects of consuming guar gum: Abdominal
   pain, diarrhea, gas, nausea (in 50 to 100 percent of people in
   high doses)[270]
Possible long-term effects of consuming guar gum: May lower
   cholesterol

Locust Bean Gum (Carob Bean Gum)
Can the human body digest this? No
Do some gut bacteria digest this? Yes
Can it alter the gut microbiome? Probably
Can it cause inflammation? Probably not
Possible immediate effects of consuming locust bean gum:
   Gastrointestinal upset in infants and young children[271]
Possible long-term effects of consuming locust bean gum:
   Unknown

Xanthan Gum
Can the human body digest this? No
Do some gut bacteria digest this? Yes
Can it alter the gut microbiome? Yes[272]
Can it cause inflammation? Probably not
Possible immediate effects of consuming xanthan gum: Diarrhea
   and gas[273]
Possible long-term effects of consuming xanthan gum: Lower
   cholesterol, lower blood sugar[274]

Inulin *(also called oligofructose, oligofructose-enriched inulin, chicory root fiber, chicory root extract, and fructooligosaccharides)*
> Can the human body digest this? No
> Do some gut bacteria digest this? Yes
> Can it alter the gut microbiome? Yes[275]
> Can it cause inflammation? Probably not
> Possible immediate effects of consuming inulin: Abdominal pain, diarrhea, gas
> Possible long-term effects of consuming inulin: Better blood sugar control, possible liver cancer[276]

Modified Food Starches
> Can the human body digest this? No
> Do some gut bacteria digest this? Yes
> Can it alter the gut microbiome? Yes[277]
> Can it cause inflammation? Probably not
> Possible immediate effects of consuming modified food starches: Diarrhea, bloating, gas[278]
> Possible long-term effects of consuming modified food starches: Unknown

Maltodextrin *(also a type of modified starch)*
> Can the human body digest this? Yes
> Do some gut bacteria digest this? Yes
> Can it alter the gut microbiome? Yes[279]
> Can it cause inflammation? Maybe
> Possible immediate effects of consuming maltodextrin: Diarrhea, bloating, gas, increased blood sugar
> Possible long-term effects of consuming maltodextrin: Necrotizing enterocolitis (bowel death) in newborns, Crohn's disease in adults[280]

Fats and Fatty Acids

Calories come in three major forms—carbohydrate, protein, and fat. The ultra-processed additives below are found in most ultra-processed foods where a fat is needed. You have probably heard of triglycerides, since that is how fats are transported around our body, and triglyceride levels measured in a standard cholesterol panel. Lecithin (this has absolutely nothing to do with lectins, which some people try to avoid—it just sounds similar), like soy lecithin, is a known cause of diarrhea, and polysorbate has been linked to weight gain.

Diglycerides and Monoglycerides

Can the human body digest this? Yes

Do some gut bacteria digest this? Probably

Can it alter the gut microbiome? Yes, but maybe not as much as other additives

Can it cause inflammation? Yes, possibly through reduction in anti-inflammatory bacteria[281]

Possible immediate effects of consuming diglycerides and monoglycerides? Unknown

Possible long-term effects of consuming diglycerides and monoglycerides? Increased cholesterol, increased blood sugar, decreased fat loss (from animal studies)[282]

Lecithins *(from soy, sunflower, or possibly something else)*

Can the human body digest this? Yes

Do some gut bacteria digest this? Possibly

Can it alter the gut microbiome? Yes,[283] but maybe not as much as other additives

Can it cause inflammation? Probably not; for colitis sufferers undergoing a flare, it is used in some meal replacements they are given when they cannot eat.

Possible immediate effects of consuming lecithins: Diarrhea, abdominal pain[284]

Possible long-term effects of consuming lecithins: Unknown

Polysorbate 60 and 80
    Can the human body digest this? Partially
    Do some gut bacteria digest this? Yes
    Can it alter the gut microbiome? Yes[285]
    Can it cause inflammation? Probably
    Possible immediate effects of consuming polysorbates: Diarrhea
    Possible long-term effects of consuming polysorbates: Colitis,
        colon cancer[286]

Polyols

These substances are mostly used as sweeteners. They have been on many lists of foods to avoid in IBS sufferers for a long time and are where the *P* in *low-FODMAP* comes from.

Glycerol/Glycerin
    Can the human body digest this? Yes
    Do some gut bacteria digest this? Yes[287]
    Can it alter the gut microbiome? Yes
    Can it cause inflammation? Probably not
    Possible immediate effects of consuming glycerol: Gas, diarrhea,
        abdominal pain (in large doses)
    Possible long-term effects of consuming glycerol: Unknown, but
        concern about possible contaminants in production[288]

Mannitol
    Can the human body digest this? Partially
    Do some gut bacteria digest this? Yes
    Can it alter the gut microbiome? Yes[289]
    Can it cause inflammation? Probably not
    Possible immediate effects of consuming mannitol: Gas,
        abdominal pain, diarrhea
    Possible long-term effects of consuming mannitol: Unknown

Sorbitol

    Can the human body digest this? Partially[290]

    Do some gut bacteria digest this? Yes

    Can it alter the gut microbiome? Yes

    Can it cause inflammation? Probably not

    Possible immediate effects of consuming sorbitol: Gas, abdominal pain[291]

    Possible long-term effects of consuming sorbitol: Unknown

Xylitol

    Can the human body digest this? Partially[292]

    Do some gut bacteria digest this? Yes

    Can it alter the gut microbiome? Yes

    Can it cause inflammation? Probably not

    Possible immediate effects of consuming xylitol: Gas, abdominal pain

    Possible long-term effects of consuming xylitol: Unknown

Not an Actual Food Category

We are eating substances that cannot be easily categorized as something the body would recognize as food (called xenobiotics), many of which aren't terribly well studied. Titanium dioxide is the exception, and enough evidence has emerged for some countries to have banned it from their food supplies.

Titanium Dioxide

    Can the human body digest this? No

    Do some gut bacteria digest this? Probably not

    Can it alter the gut microbiome? Unknown

    Can it cause gut inflammation? Yes[293]

    Possible immediate effect of consuming titanium dioxide: Unknown

    Possible long-term effects of consuming titanium dioxide: Worsening of IBD,[294] potential cancer-causing substance[295]

Appendix B

A Week of Eating Everything (Real)

In real life, cooking can be a harried affair, especially on weekdays, but also during weekends when there are kids' sporting events to attend and birthday parties to drive to. The following relatively simple schedule assumes that you have the weekend off from work and no older relatives to care for or other significant weekend obligations. That's a big assumption given how many jobs require night hours and weekends. So consider this just one example—and if something else works better for you, do that!

Day 1—This would be a Sunday for me, but it may not be for you. Ideally, it's a day off before the busyness of the week begins. Plan for something quick and easy since this is also grocery shopping (or ordering!) day. Check out the baked salmon recipes in Appendix C and consider pairing with a quick side of couscous and roasted veggies or a simple green salad with a homemade dressing you can use during the rest of the week. Or google fifteen-minute meals, but give yourself thirty minutes if it is only your first or second time making the dish.

Day 2— This is a cooking night. The fridge is full of just-purchased ingredients, so you might as well put them to good use. But whatever you make, be sure to have enough for the next day. Consider the grilled chicken recipe in Appendix C and pair with pasta and a jarred, additive-free sauce. If you made a lot of roasted veggies on Day 1, serve them as well.

Day 3—Leftovers from cooking night. Fewer dishes. Yay!

Day 4 (this is Wednesday for me)—This is slow cooker recipe day. You can buy a simple slow cooker for around twenty dollars or spring for a fancy Instant Pot, which is around one hundred dollars. Instant Pots take some getting used to. Slow cookers are fairly straightforward. Buy a large slow cooker if you are feeding a family, and make enough for two nights.

It's midweek and things are possibly getting tougher organization-wise. I prefer recipes that can be thrown together in the morning and left for eight to ten hours so dinner is ready to go at the end of the day. Consider making a big batch of chili. There's a recipe in Appendix C. Pair with a salad and some of the dressing from Day 1 if you've made that. If you haven't, while the chili is staying warm, consider throwing together a quick dressing (the lemon-pepper dressing in Appendix C would be awesome here).

Day 5—Leftovers from slow cooker night. Leftovers are the best time-saver of all!

Day 6 (this is Friday for me)—Congratulations! You've just spent nearly a week putting together meals. Feel free to put together another and enjoy the leftovers on Day 7, or give yourself the night off. Try to order out from a place that you know has the fewest gut-roiling additives. See chapter 12 for tips.

Day 7—This is pre-shopping day. I try to use up the ingredients left in the fridge before they go bad. Consider making the japchae from Appendix C. While the recipe calls for specific veggies, substitutions are allowed and encouraged!

Now that you know what you are making, it's time to put together your grocery list. You can use an app if you are into the electronic thing (apps can remember lists if you keep to a certain pattern, which may save time). If you prefer paper, copy the alphabetical list of additives to avoid in Appendix A for a quick reference guide. So plan, but plan to be less than perfect. The key to eating everything again is to use processed foods to your advantage to avoid eating the ultra-processed stuff.

Appendix C

Twenty-Five
Real-Food Recipes

Bread and Bread Alternatives

Einkorn Focaccia Bread
Makes one focaccia to feed 6–8 • Takes 2 hours 30 minutes
accounting for rising time

If you want to bake an easy bread at home, the eminent Dr. Peter Lio, home baker extraordinaire and clinical assistant professor of dermatology at Northwestern University, has graciously shared his recipe. Dr. Lio recommends using einkorn flour made from an older strain of cultivated wheat, which helps him with digestion and might be easier for those with gluten sensitivity (note, einkorn still contains some gluten so this recipe is *not* for those suffering with celiac disease). If you do not have ready access to einkorn flour, all-purpose flour can be substituted.

Ingredients
2 cups filtered warm water (around 110°F)
1 tablespoon granulated white sugar
1 teaspoon yeast

5 cups einkorn flour (or all-purpose flour if that's what you have),
plus some extra for dusting

2 teaspoons kosher salt, divided

3 tablespoons extra-virgin olive oil, plus more for greasing

Steps

1. Combine the water and sugar in a bowl (use an electric mixer if you have it) and sprinkle the yeast on top. Set aside and allow the yeast to become foamy, which it will do in about 5 minutes. If it doesn't, either your water was too hot and killed the yeast, or the yeast is no longer active, so you will need to start over with new water, sugar, and yeast.

2. In a separate bowl, whisk the flour with 1½ teaspoons of the salt. Add one-quarter of the flour at a time to the water-and-yeast mixture while beating with the dough hook attachment to bring together in a firm dough. If you don't have a stand mixer, mix with a spatula until it begins to come together and then use your hands to finish forming the mixture into a dough.

3. Remove the dough from the mixer and place it into a bowl with a light coating of oil. Cover it with a kitchen towel and allow it to rise for about 45 minutes or until approximately doubled in size.

4. Turn the dough out onto a clean work surface that has been lightly floured. Fold the dough in half four times and place it back into the bowl. Cover it with the towel and allow it to rise another 45 minutes.

5. Preheat the oven to 500°F (or to 450°F on the convection setting).

6. Drizzle 3 tablespoons of extra-virgin olive oil onto the bottom of a 8 × 11–inch high-sided baking dish.

7. Divide the dough in half and press out one-half of the dough to completely and evenly cover the dish (you can freeze the other half or bake it afterward).

8. Sprinkle the remaining ½ teaspoon of salt evenly over the top.

9. Bake for about 17 minutes until lightly browned, rotating it 180 degrees after 10 minutes for even browning. Allow the focaccia to cool slightly before enjoying.

Seriously Good Homemade Tortillas

Makes 6 approximately 8-inch tortillas • Takes about 1 hour,
including dough resting time

As noted in chapter 6, soft store-bought tortillas are often full of additives to keep them that way. But sometimes you just don't want a crunchy taco shell. So you have a choice: you can chance it with the store-bought tortillas (the frozen ones may not have the softening additives, so try those first), or you can make your own. My son's friend describes these as heaven. And who am I to argue? But heaven takes some time, so I generally make these when I have leftovers on hand so I don't have to make a bunch of other things while making the tortillas. Another option is to throw some chicken in a slow cooker or Instant Pot and then focus on your tortillas. However you manage it, these are worth your time.

Ingredients
2 cups all-purpose flour, plus some extra for dusting
½ teaspoon baking powder
½ teaspoon salt
3 tablespoons cold unsalted butter
¾ cup warm water
1 teaspoon oil (any kind is fine)

Steps
1. Combine the flour, baking powder, and salt in a medium or large bowl and mix well.
2. Add butter in small pats and work it into the flour with your fingers until the butter is well incorporated and the mixture looks like small pebbles. You can also do this with an electric hand mixer on low speed.
3. Add the water and mix with a fork until the dough almost comes together. Put some flour on your hands and give the dough a few kneads in the bowl until a ball is formed. You should always feel free to add a little more water if the dough is dry and not coming together or a little more flour if the dough is wet or too sticky to work with. Alternatively, you could add the

water on low speed using your electric mixer and turn it off when you see the dough start to come together.

4. Remove the dough from the bowl and place it on a lightly floured clean counter or cutting board. Use your hands to form a thick rope with the dough, about 15 inches long. Cut the dough into six pieces. Form each piece into a small ball.

5. Brush the oil on the dough balls so they don't dry out. Cover them with plastic wrap and allow them to rest for 30 minutes.

6. When you are ready to get going, heat a cast-iron skillet (or whatever heavy skillet you own) on medium-high for several minutes.

7. Flour your counter or cutting board and a rolling pin (small rolling pins work better, but anything will do). Roll the balls out to circles 6 to 8 inches in diameter (you won't get perfect circles unless you invest in a tortilla press, but you can come close by rolling and rotating the pin 45 degrees with each push).

8. Reduce the heat to medium. Place one rolled out tortilla into the hot skillet. When bubbles start to form on the top, flip the tortilla and cook for about 30 seconds more. (If you notice the tortillas are burning, reduce the heat further.) Remove the tortilla onto a plate that you cover to keep the tortillas warm and repeat with the remaining balls.

9. Enjoy the praise your family will bestow upon you for providing them with a piece of heaven.

Arepas
Serves 4-6 • Takes 30 minutes

Arepas are small, savory corn cakes especially popular in Colombian and Venezuelan cuisine. They're kind of like thick pancakes that can be used as a bread substitute. I discovered this Latin American staple in high school at a Miami festival called Calle Ocho, named after a famous street in the Little Havana neighborhood. The festival celebrates Latin American culture. I had been recruited by a friend to sell frozen lemonade from a cart. My cart was fortuitously placed next to an arepa cart. With the fragrant fried smell wafting over and the lemonade money burning a hole in my pocket, I bought a simple cheese-filled arepa. It was pretty wonderful. This is my interpretation of that—with credit to my daughter's friend Alexandra, who shared her grandmother's technique with me.

Ingredients
2 cups masarepa cornmeal (see notes)
½ teaspoon salt
2¼ cups water
Vegetable oil for frying
Slices of your favorite firm cheese for filling (see notes)

Steps
1. Preheat the oven to 325°F.
2. In a medium bowl, mix the masarepa and salt. Then add the water and mix with your fingers until the lumps are gone. The dough should be wet but not sticking easily to your fingers. Allow it to rest for 5 minutes.
3. Divide the dough into eight equal portions. Moisten your hands with water and roll one portion into a small ball about the size of an orange, then use your palms to gently flatten it into a ½-inch-thick disk, keeping it as circular as possible. Repeat with the remaining dough.
4. Heat a thin layer of oil in a nonstick or cast-iron skillet on medium-high heat. When very hot, add the arepas, frying four at a time (or as many will fit in your skillet without overcrowding). Cook for 3 to 4 minutes per side or until well browned and crispy on the outside.
5. Place the arepas on a baking sheet and bake in the oven for another 10 minutes.
6. When cool enough to handle, slice open the arepas longitudinally and place the cheese inside. Put them back in the oven for another 2 minutes to melt the cheese.

Notes: Masarepa is precooked ground corn flour that can be purchased in the international aisles of supermarkets, in Latin food markets, or online. There is no substitute for this ingredient. The man making the arepas at Calle Ocho made them a bit thinner, adding the cheese and topping with another finished arepa, and then wrapping it in foil to create an easy grab-and-go item. The heat from the just-fried arepas immediately wrapped in foil melted the cheese all on its own. You can do this, too, if you need to speed up the process and have a quick to-go breakfast or lunch. I like to fill my arepas with muenster slices because my kids like it, and we always have some on hand, but use whatever firm cheese you like. Consider adding other fillings (google Venezuelan arepas for some ideas) as arepas work well as a gluten-free sandwich option if you are avoiding wheat-based foods.

Breakfast

Perfect Breakfast Granola
Serves about 15 • Takes approximately 1 hour

This granola makes it incredibly easy to avoid commercially made breakfast cereals. If you are also trying to avoid gluten, gluten-free oats are readily available in most supermarkets and specialty stores. This recipe makes about two large mason jars' worth of granola (with some left over for you to enjoy while the granola cools!). Don't have the exact ingredients? Feel free to improvise with your favorite dried fruits and nuts. Almost anything works in this recipe. Just remember to keep the fruit out of the oven and add it at the end when everything else has cooled.

Ingredients
5 cups old-fashioned rolled oats
1 heaping cup sliced almonds
1 heaping cup pecan pieces or halves
3 packed tablespoons brown sugar
½ teaspoon cinnamon (or more if you like cinnamon)
¼ cup vegetable oil
¼ cup maple syrup (see note)
½ teaspoon salt
½ cup raisins
½ cup dried cranberries

Steps
1. Preheat the oven to 250°F. Arrange one rack about one-third of the way from the bottom and another rack one-third of the way from the top.
2. Combine the oats, almonds, pecans, brown sugar, and cinnamon in a large bowl. Mix well to make sure the brown sugar is evenly distributed.
3. In a small bowl or liquid measuring cup, combine the oil and syrup. Add the salt and give it a few stirs to mix.

4. Pour the wet mixture onto the dry ingredients and mix well to moisten all the oats.
5. Spread the granola onto two rimmed baking sheets.
6. Bake for 45 minutes, stirring the granola and switching the baking sheets top to bottom every 15 minutes until the granola is dry and toasted to your liking.
7. Allow the granola to cool on the baking sheets, then mix in the raisins and cranberries until the fruit is well distributed. Store in sealed containers. Granola will last for about a week stored at room temperature—though in my house, it's usually gone in a few days!—or for a few weeks in the fridge.

Note: To keep this homemade granola additive-free, I recommend using pure maple syrup.

Ridiculously Easy Pancakes
Serves 3–4 • Takes 15 minutes

I love this recipe because I can remember it. It's so easy, you will wonder why you ever bought the mix. Make a double batch if you want to freeze some to reheat for a quick breakfast later in the week.

Ingredients
1 cup flour
1 tablespoon white or light brown sugar
1 tablespoon baking powder
½ teaspoon salt
1 cup milk
1 large or extra-large egg, beaten
2 tablespoons vegetable oil
Unsalted butter for cooking

Steps

1. In a large mixing bowl, whisk together (or use an electric mixer) the flour, sugar, baking powder, salt, milk, egg, and oil until well combined. Different recipes will give you a different order for adding things together. It's early. Who cares? If the batter is too thin, add another tablespoon or two of flour. If it's too thick, add a tablespoon or two of milk.
2. Heat a nonstick skillet over medium heat. Throw in a pat of butter and swirl it around the skillet to coat, letting it heat until just bubbling.
3. Add ¼ to ⅓ cupfuls of pancake batter depending on how big you like your pancakes. Let the batter cook until it's bubbling on top and the edges look brownish, then flip the pancakes and cook for another few minutes until browned on the other side. Repeat until all the batter is used up.

Dan's Breakfast Smoothies

I took my husband's cousin, Dan, to a vegan restaurant some years ago mainly because he's a vegan, and back then I had no idea what to feed him. He hated it, although he was trying to look like he didn't. He calmly (he's always very calm, maybe a side effect of veganism?) explained to me that *vegan* doesn't necessarily mean healthy. What I didn't appreciate at the time was the amount of ultra-processed food that restaurant was serving. If you're doing a plant-based diet, the key is to stick with actual plants, not packets.

Dan is a pretty buff guy and needs to eat a lot. I've seen him make a smoothie from a counter full of fruits and veggies. He does a lot of smoothies for a quick energy fix. I figured if anyone knows how to make a great smoothie, it's Dan. Here are a couple of his best. Smoothies are a perfect way to use up too-soft berries or other fruit that no one ate the previous week. Add a teaspoon or two of chia seeds after you've blended it for a little extra protein if you like that sort of thing.

Honeydew and Mint Smoothie
Serves 2–3 • Takes 5 minutes

Ingredients
Half or a whole honeydew melon, seeded and cubed

3 mint leaves

Steps
1. In a blender, blend the melon and mint together until smooth.
2. Pour it into two or three glasses and serve right away. Now you have a cool way to start your day.

Banana, Date, and Berry Smoothie (with some veggies, but don't be scared)
Serves 2–3 • Takes 5 minutes

Ingredients
2 bananas

1 cup fresh or frozen berries of your choice

2 celery stalks sliced into ¼-inch pieces

2 pitted Medjool dates

½ cup water

Steps
1. In a blender, combine the bananas, berries, celery, dates, and water, and blend it all together until smooth.
2. Pour it into two or three glasses and serve right away.

Mains

___

Simple Grilled Chicken
Serves 4–6 • Takes 20 minutes (not including marinating time)

The first step to making really good grilled chicken that cooks up quickly is buying thinly sliced cutlets. If you can't find these, you can slice them thinly yourself. Plant your nondominant hand on top of a boneless, skinless chicken breast, applying pressure so the breast doesn't move. Use a good chef's knife to cut it horizontally down the center so you wind up with two thinner pieces. (When you get pretty good at this, you can get a large boneless, skinless breast to cut into thirds.) This cooks up really quickly and evenly and is a great weeknight go-to.

The second step to making good grilled chicken is to marinate it for even just 15 minutes in something acidic. It helps white meat from becoming tough when you cook it. This holds true for making any kind of chicken. Indian cooking usually calls for a yogurt marinade, fried chicken mavens usually marinate in a buttermilk mix, but I prefer good old lemon juice since I usually have lemons on hand. If you don't have time to marinate, that's okay, too, just watch your cook time and be careful not to overcook the chicken.

Ingredients
1 lemon, juiced
3 tablespoons olive oil
½ teaspoon kosher salt
¼ teaspoon ground black pepper
2 pounds thinly sliced chicken cutlets
Canola or grapeseed oil for grilling (see note)

Steps
1. Combine the lemon juice, olive oil, salt, and pepper in a medium-sized bowl. Add the chicken cutlets, turning to coat. Marinate for 15 minutes or up to several hours. (If you are going to leave it to marinate for more than

15 minutes, cover with plastic wrap and pop it in the fridge to keep it from spoiling.)

2. Brush a grill pan or an outside grill with an oil that has a high-temperature smoke point (like canola or grapeseed oil). Heat until very hot (using hot pans is the best pro tip I ever got) over medium-high heat on the stove or high heat on the grill.

3. Remove the chicken from the marinade. Put the chicken on the pan or grill, cover it with a stockpot cover if using your stove or with the grill cover if outside, and cook it until the edges start to look like they are browning (3–5 minutes depending on the thickness—you can peek as often as you like until you get a sense for the timing). Flip the chicken and cook for an additional 3–5 minutes. Flip again if necessary to make sure it's nicely browned.

4. You can check for doneness by making a small cut in the chicken to make sure the juices run clear or by using a meat thermometer, which should register at 165°F.

Variations: You can spice things up by sprinkling the breasts with chili powder or whatever spices you like before you grill them. If you have an additive-free BBQ sauce, make this into a BBQ night by brushing some on just before the chicken is done (if you do this too soon, the sugar in it will burn before the chicken is cooked, so wait until the end).

Oven "Fried" Chicken
Serves 4-6 • Takes 30 minutes

Frying is messy and time-consuming, so if we can eat less fried foods, why not? This is my go-to recipe for "fried" chicken at home. And I'll be honest, it isn't the same as actual fried chicken (nothing is), but with extra savory flavor from the Parmesan cheese in the breading, it's a pretty good substitute—and it's quick with an easy cleanup. (To avoid additives, shred your own cheese from a block of Parmesan. It takes 2 minutes, and it's worth it!)

Ingredients

Canola or grapeseed oil for greasing

2 cups additive-free bread crumbs (see notes)

½ cup thinly shredded Parmesan

2 teaspoons dried Italian seasoning (see notes)

½ teaspoon kosher salt

¼ teaspoon ground black pepper

2 pounds thinly sliced chicken cutlets (see notes)

3 tablespoons unsalted butter, melted

Steps

1. Preheat the oven to 425°F (or to 375°F on the convection setting). Lightly brush a baking sheet with a high-heat oil such as canola or grapeseed.

2. Mix the bread crumbs with the cheese, Italian seasoning, salt, and pepper in a flat bowl or baking dish.

3. Generously brush a piece of chicken on both sides with some of the melted butter and then drop it into the bread crumb mixture to coat both sides well. Place the coated chicken onto the baking sheet and repeat with all the pieces of chicken.

4. Bake the chicken until the breading is nicely browned and the chicken is fully cooked (about 20 minutes depending on the thickness of the chicken). To check for doneness, use a meat thermometer, which should register 165°F, or remove a test piece onto a plate and cut it to see if the juices run clear.

Variation: After 15 minutes of cooking, top the chicken breasts with a tablespoon of tomato sauce and a slice of fresh mozzarella. Bake for an additional 5 minutes or until the cheese is nice and bubbly and the chicken is cooked through.

Notes: If you can't find thinly sliced chicken cutlets, cut your own from boneless skinless chicken breast. See the Simple Grilled Chicken recipe, page 211, for directions. If you can't find regular bread crumbs that are additive-free, try looking for additive-free panko (Ingredients in the Kikkoman brand are just flour, sugar, yeast, and salt, and these crunchy crumbs work great). If you don't have Italian seasoning on hand, make your own with equal parts dried oregano, basil, thyme, rosemary, parsley, and garlic powder, or whichever of those herbs you have on hand. It's all good. If you try to cut a piece of chicken to check it while it's still on the pan, the juices will run out and ruin the crispy crust on the other pieces. So even though it might seem fussy, test your chicken on a separate plate.

Slow Cooker Chicken Tacos
Serves 4–6 • Takes 8 hours in the slow cooker
plus 5 minutes prep time

This is the best quick weeknight dinner. The chicken may take 8 hours in the slow cooker, but only a few minutes of active prep time (not including the time it takes to prep your toppings) is needed. So if you don't have a slow cooker, think about getting one. They're inexpensive and great for set-it-and-forget-it meals like this.

Ingredients
2 pounds boneless, skinless chicken breast (see note)
1 jar of your favorite additive-free salsa
Salt and pepper to taste
Hard corn tortillas or additive-free soft tortillas (recipe on page 203 or
  store-bought)

Topping ideas:
Shredded lettuce
Diced tomatoes
Sliced sweet red peppers
Shredded Colby jack cheese
Chopped fresh cilantro
Lime wedges for squeezing
Sour cream without additives (we love the Daisy brand)
Guacamole (recipe on page 228 or store-bought)

Steps

1. Combine the chicken and salsa in a slow cooker. Cover and cook on low for 6 to 8 hours.
2. Shred the chicken with two forks and let it sit in the sauce for a few minutes before serving. Taste and add a little salt and pepper if you think it needs a little more seasoning.
3. Serve the chicken in taco shells or tortillas with whatever toppings you like.

Note: You can make this with leftover cooked chicken (such as my Simple Grilled Chicken, page 211) or the meat from an additive-free rotisserie chicken. Simply shred the cooked chicken, then place it into a medium saucepan and add the salsa. Heat on medium for 5 minutes or until the chicken is nice and warm. If you're using my chicken recipe, consider marinating it in lime juice instead of lemon, and definitely add the optional chili powder.

Learning to Love Your Slow Cooker Chili
Serves 4–6 • Takes 8 hours in the slow cooker
plus 20 minutes prep time

If chicken tacos don't convince you to buy a slow cooker, perhaps this chili will. It's a great busy day go-to and very forgiving time-wise: If you need to go to work for longer, the chili can go for 9 hours, or if you have hungry people clamoring for dinner sooner, 6 hours is fine. It's also a family favorite dish. I've been asked for this recipe by friends whose kids go home raving about it!

Ingredients
1½ pounds ground beef (see note)
1 yellow onion, diced
1 bell pepper (any color), diced
1 (28-ounce) can crushed tomatoes
3 (14-ounce) cans garbanzo, cannellini, and red beans (or any combination), drained and rinsed

1 teaspoon to 1 tablespoon chili powder (depending on your spice preference)

1½ teaspoons cumin

1½ teaspoons sweet or smoked paprika

1 teaspoon garlic powder

½ teaspoon salt

½ teaspoon oregano

¼ teaspoon ground black pepper

½ to 1 cup water

Steps

1. Heat a large skillet over medium-high heat. Brown the ground beef, breaking it up with a spoon as it cooks (see note). Drain the fat.
2. Combine the beef, onion, pepper, tomatoes, beans, chili powder, cumin, paprika, garlic powder, salt, oregano, and pepper in your slow cooker. Add ½ to 1 cup of water to the tomato can, swirl it around, and then add it to the slow cooker to thin out the chili a bit—use less water if you like a thicker chili. Mix all the ingredients well.
3. Cover and cook on low for 6 to 8 hours. (A little longer won't hurt it, either.)

Note: If you use lean ground beef, such as 90/10 beef, you may need to cook it in some canola or grapeseed oil to prevent it from sticking to the pan. Beef with a higher fat ratio does not need additional oil.

Salmon with Bruschetta Topping
Serves 3–4 • Takes 15 minutes

I'll admit that I'm not the best fish chef, but salmon is hard to mess up. It is also extremely healthy—not just for your gut, but probably for your heart and brain, too. And sure, you can use a cast-iron skillet and crisp the skin and do lots of fancy things to it, but you don't have to. This is one of those recipes that looks like you spent a lot of time on it when you really didn't. The bruschetta topping can be made in advance or while the salmon is cooking. Double the tomato topping recipe to have extra on hand to put on toasted bread that day or the next.

Ingredients

1–1½ pounds salmon, cut into 3–4 pieces
1 tablespoon olive oil
Salt to taste
Ground black pepper to taste
2 ripe plum tomatoes, diced
½ yellow onion, finely diced
1 garlic clove, crushed or minced
1 tablespoon thinly sliced fresh basil leaves
1 teaspoon balsamic vinegar

Steps

1. Heat the oven on a high broil for 10 minutes. Line a rimmed sheet pan with aluminum foil.
2. Rub your salmon with the olive oil and season with salt and pepper. Place it on the sheet pan. Broil on the middle rack for about 10 minutes until the fish starts to lightly brown on top.
3. While the salmon is cooking, prepare the bruschetta topping. Combine the tomatoes, onion, garlic, basil, and balsamic vinegar in a small bowl.
4. When the salmon is starting to brown a little, remove it from the oven and spoon the bruschetta on top.
5. Turn off the oven and return the topped fish to the oven for a minute or two to warm everything up.

Moroccan Salmon
Serves 3–4 • Takes 15 minutes

If the bruschetta topping is too much work, this is an even simpler way to get a flavorful fish dish on the table fast. This also works well with whatever fish you might have on hand. If you are working with thin fillets, don't broil them but use a 400°F oven and watch the fish carefully as it may not need a full 10 minutes to cook. If the fillets are thicker, they may need a little more time. Fish should flake easily with a fork when fully cooked. Broil it for 1–2 minutes at the end to get some nice color.

Ingredients
1–1½ pounds salmon, cut into 3–4 pieces
1 tablespoon olive oil
½ teaspoon ras el hanout seasoning (see note)
Salt and pepper to taste
1 lemon

Steps
1. Heat oven on broil for 10 minutes. Line a sheet pan with aluminum foil.
2. Rub your salmon with olive oil and season it with ras el hanout, salt, and pepper. Place it on the sheet pan. Broil on the middle rack for about 10 minutes until the fish starts to lightly brown on top.
3. Cut the lemon in half. Cut one of the halves into thin slices. Reserve the other half.
4. When the fish is slightly browning on top, remove it from the oven and top it with the lemon slices.
5. Return the fish to the broiler for 1–2 minutes. The lemon slices should get slightly browned. Remove it from the oven and squeeze lemon juice over the fish.

Note: Ras el hanout is a fragrant spice blend originating in Morocco, Algeria, and Tunisia. There are different formulations, but it's often made from cumin, coriander, cinnamon, ginger, pepper, and turmeric. If you don't have it, any other style seasoning mix you like can work well here, too—even just chili powder gives things a nice kick.

Cacio e Pepe (AKA Italian Mac 'n' Cheese)
Serves 4 • Takes 20 minutes

When we visited Rome, we were introduced to a dish called cacio e pepe (or cheese and pepper). My kids immediately identified this as a fancy mac 'n' cheese dish. Even better, the whole family loved it, so I decided to try making it at home. After learning the hard way that you absolutely must put the sauce together in exactly the order called for, I made a successful cacio e pepe. It's easy, it's quick, it's totally delicious, and everyone eats it. This may take a couple of attempts to get right, but don't despair! Learning to make a butter or olive oil–based sauce using pasta water as a binder is a neat cooking trick and one worth learning if you like Italian food.

Ingredients
Salt, to taste
3 tablespoons unsalted butter
¾ teaspoon ground black pepper, more for garnish
1 (8-ounce) package dried egg fettuccini (see note)
1 cup fresh, thinly shredded Parmesan cheese, divided
½ cup fresh, thinly shredded pecorino Romano cheese

Steps
1. Bring a large pot of water to a boil (add salt to the water to taste—the Italians do!).
2. Melt the butter in a large sauté pan on medium-low heat (make sure the pan is big enough to hold your pasta, which you will be adding later). As the butter is melting, add the pepper and give it a stir. When the butter has completely melted, turn off the heat.
3. Add your pasta to the water and cook per the package directions. Just before the pasta is done, remove one cup of pasta water from the pot. (This stuff is magical! Pasta water has the starch from the pasta and is a great binder for so many Italian sauces.) Set the pasta water aside and drain your pasta.

4. Turn the heat back on low under your butter-pepper mixture and add about half of the pasta water. Then carefully add your pasta, giving it a quick coat in the mixture using tongs.
5. Add ¾ cup Parmesan cheese and mix it around with the tongs to incorporate.
6. Turn the heat off and add the pecorino Romano cheese, incorporating with tongs until well melted. If things are too clumpy, add more of the pasta water until your sauce is the consistency you want. Do this slowly so as not to thin it out too much.
7. Garnish with more pepper and the remaining ¼ cup Parmesan cheese.

Note: Use whatever pasta you like. I like using egg fettucine because the egg in the pasta gives it a little richness, and the sauce clings nicely to thicker noodles.

Japchae (Korean Noodles with Vegetables)
Serves 4–6 • Takes 30 minutes

One winter, a Korean Canadian friend from medical school wanted a place to vacation with his family. So we opened our Florida home to our friend and his wife and kids, his siblings, and, most importantly, his parents. Our friend's mother and her daughter-in-law began cooking up a storm in the kitchen. My husband quietly asked to join them. By the end of the week, he could make a handful of Korean dishes pretty authentically. This one has become a family favorite. You can make it heartier by adding sliced grilled beef that has been well seasoned—rib eye and sirloin work well. Add the beef at the end, just before serving. If you like a little heat, serve it with a side of kimchi (spicy fermented cabbage, available in lots of grocery stores these days or in Asian markets, which sometimes make it in-house)—a wonderful source of real probiotics!

Ingredients

12 ounces dried sweet potato noodles (see notes)

For the stir-fried vegetables:
2 tablespoons vegetable oil
2 zucchini or yellow squash (or one of each), julienned
2 carrots, julienned
1 red bell pepper, thinly sliced
½ medium or large red onion, thinly sliced
Handful of sliced shiitake mushrooms (see notes)
¼ teaspoon ground white pepper
¼ teaspoon garlic powder
¼ teaspoon onion powder
¼ teaspoon salt
3 garlic cloves, minced

For the noodles:
2 tablespoons sesame oil
1–2 tablespoons brown sugar (depending on how sweet you like it)
1 teaspoon onion powder
1 teaspoon garlic powder
1–2 tablespoons soy sauce (depending on how salty you like it)
1 teaspoon toasted sesame seeds

Steps
1. Prepare the noodles according to the package directions until they are chewy but not mushy. Drain. Immediately rinse with cold water to stop the cooking process. Set aside.
2. For the vegetables: Heat a wok or large sauté pan over medium-high heat until very hot. Pour in the vegetable oil and reduce the heat to medium. Cook the zucchini, carrots, bell pepper, and onion until softened, about 4–5 minutes, stirring frequently. As the vegetables are cooking, add the

white pepper, garlic and onion powders, and salt. Stir in the fresh or presoaked and drained mushrooms.

3. Add the minced garlic and cook one more minute until fragrant. Remove the vegetables from the wok and set aside.

4. For the noodles: Return the wok to medium heat and pour in the sesame oil. Add the cooked noodles and toss to coat. Add the sugar (starting with 1 tablespoon), onion powder, and garlic powder and stir well to coat. Add the soy sauce (starting with 1 tablespoon) and taste. Adjust the flavor with more sugar and soy sauce as desired.

5. Return the veggies to the wok and mix well. Top with sesame seeds and serve.

Notes: The noodles you'll need for this dish are sometimes sold as glass noodles or Korean vermicelli. Check the ingredients; only sweet potato should be listed. You can use fresh or dried shiitake. Soak the dried mushrooms in a bowl of water to rehydrate before using.

Sides and Snacks

Baingan Bharta
Serves 4–6 • Takes 40 minutes

This is my attempt at recreating my favorite eggplant dish of all time. Several friends with Indian heritage have tried to teach me how to make various Indian dishes over the years. This recipe is the culmination of their efforts. However, I am in no way an Indian food chef. It is one recipe, and if you like it, you should definitely try some dishes made by actual Indian chefs. Or better yet, get an Indian food cookbook and try out a bunch of dishes yourself. The vegetarian options, if you are going that route with your diet, are pretty much endless! One helpful trick for making this recipe: the eggplant needs about 30 minutes in the oven, so you can chop the other ingredients while it's roasting. Your eggplant should be just about done when you are on step 5. This will allow a few minutes for the eggplant to cool before step 6.

Ingredients
1½ tablespoons olive oil or other mild-flavored oil, divided
1 large or 2 medium eggplants
1 yellow onion, diced
2 garlic cloves, minced
1 (1-inch) piece fresh ginger, peeled and grated
1 teaspoon cumin
1 teaspoon turmeric
½ teaspoon garam masala
½ teaspoon salt
1 large tomato or 2 plum tomatoes, diced
½ cup frozen peas, thawed
Handful of cilantro, roughly chopped

Steps

1. Preheat the oven to 425°F (or to 375°F on the convection setting).
2. Line a baking sheet with foil and pour a ½ tablespoon of oil onto the foil. Coat evenly with a pastry brush.
3. Slice the eggplant in half longitudinally and place it cut side down on the oil-coated baking sheet. Roast until very soft when the skin is pressed, about 30 minutes. The cut side should be nicely browned.
4. Heat a tablespoon of oil in a large sauté pan on medium heat.
5. Add the onion and cook until translucent on low heat, approximately 10 minutes. Then add the garlic and ginger and cook until fragrant, about a minute more.
6. Add the cumin, turmeric, garam masala, and salt, and mix well. Then add the tomatoes and cook until well softened, about 5 to 10 minutes. If the mixture starts to dry out, add a tablespoon or two of water.
7. While your tomatoes are cooking down, cut the top off the eggplant and peel it. Mash the eggplant with a potato masher and add it to the sauté pan. Mix well. Taste and adjust the spices to your liking.
8. Add the peas and cook on low for another 5 minutes. When it's ready to serve, top it with chopped cilantro.

Fun with Fruit Salad
Serves 4 • Takes 10 minutes

Fruit is a great way of getting fiber into our diets without the additives. The problem with fruit is that it needs to be washed and cut up if you have kids or want something easier to eat, and it doesn't last long once you've sliced it. This fruit salad can be eaten right away but also can be kept in the fridge for a day or so due to the addition of a bit of lemon juice. The cinnamon adds a little something to keep things interesting. Use the fruits suggested below or whatever you have on hand. Like smoothies (page 209-210), it's a great way to get rid of fruit that needs to be eaten before it goes off. To make this more of a dessert, you can serve it with whipped cream (page 234-235).

Ingredients

1 red apple, cut into bite-size pieces
1 pear, cut into bite-size pieces
1 cup grapes, sliced in half if you have the time
1 cup strawberries, sliced in half if small, into quarters if bigger
1 cup blueberries
1 cup raspberries
½ lemon, juiced
¼ teaspoon ground cinnamon

Steps

Mix the apple, pear, grapes, strawberries, blueberries, and raspberries in a large bowl or container with a lid. Sprinkle the lemon juice and cinnamon on top and give it a good stir to distribute evenly. Cover and store for a day or so in the refrigerator if you're not eating it immediately.

Quick Side Dish Ideas

Rice: Making rice in a dedicated rice cooker or Instant Pot is definitely the way to go. Perfect rice, easy cleanup.

Couscous: I love this side almost more than any other food. Boil 1 cup of chicken broth with a little butter and a pinch of salt and pepper. Turn off the heat, add 1 cup of couscous, cover, and you have a side dish in 5 minutes with minimal labor. Add some other herbs if you want. There really is nothing better.

Roasting veggies: There's no excuse not to make vegetables taste good. If you grew up in a home where people boiled vegetables, I understand your pain. So did I. You can break the chain. So many kinds of vegetables can be roasted, though this works best with heartier vegetables. Heat your oven to 425°F (or to 375°F on the convection setting). Take eggplant, zucchini, broccoli, cauliflower, sweet peppers, or other vegetables of your choice and cut them into ½-inch to 1-inch cubes. Place them on an oiled baking tray, or one lined with parchment paper for easier cleanup, and drizzle a bit more olive oil over them. Sprinkle them with salt and pepper and roast for about 10 minutes or until brown. Flip them with a spatula and roast for another 5 minutes or until the other side begins to brown.

Whatever you can't roast, stir fry. Heat up a little olive oil in a wok or sauté pan, add a crushed garlic clove or two, and allow it to get fragrant (about 30 seconds). Add your intended vegetables (let's say green beans), salt and pepper to taste, mix it up, add 1 or 2 tablespoons of water, cover, and steam for a few minutes until desired tenderness.

Dressings and Dips

Creamy Lemon-Pepper Dressing
Makes approximately 1 cup of dressing • Takes 5 minutes

This versatile creamy dressing most closely resembles a Caesar dressing and would resemble it more if you added a bit of Parmesan cheese. It goes great with almost any type of salad and also works as a dip (just use more additive-free mayo to thicken it up).

Ingredients
½ cup additive-free mayonnaise
1 tablespoon Dijon mustard
1 garlic clove, minced (see note)
1 lemon, juiced
⅛ teaspoon ground black pepper
Pinch of salt

Steps
Put the mayo, mustard, garlic, lemon juice, pepper, and salt into a bowl or jar. Beat with a fork until the ingredients are well blended and it has a smooth consistency. Taste and adjust salt and pepper as you like. Serve right away or store tightly covered in the fridge for up to a week.

Note: Take out the sprout in the center of the garlic clove before you mince, particularly if it is turning green. It can impart a bitter flavor, and a chef in Italy suggested to me that it is harder to digest.

Lemon-Garlic Vinaigrette
Makes approximately 1 cup of dressing • Takes 5 minutes

This dressing goes well with Greek salad or any other salad where a garlicky, lemony tang is desired. This recipe has several items in common with the creamy dressing above, so you'll quickly notice that keeping lemons and fresh garlic on hand provides you with lots of meal prep options.

Ingredients
½ cup extra-virgin olive oil
2 garlic cloves, minced
1 tablespoon white wine or red vinegar
1 lemon, juiced
¼ teaspoon dried oregano
Pinch of salt
Pinch of ground black pepper

Steps
Put the olive oil, garlic, vinegar, lemon juice, oregano, salt, and pepper in a bowl or jar. Beat with a fork until the ingredients are well blended and the oil has emulsified. Taste and adjust salt and pepper as you like. Serve right away or store tightly covered in the fridge for up to a week (since there are no emulsifiers, you will have to give it a quick shake or stir to re-emulsify).

Family Favorite Guacamole
Serves 1–6 depending on if my daughter is there • Takes 10 minutes

This is a flavorful guacamole concocted by my husband (who is actually the chef in the family) to re-create our favorite restaurant guac. When I make guacamole, I just mash an avocado and add lime juice, salt, and cilantro if I have it. You can do this, too. It's a perfectly fine guacamole. However, the kids vote for my husband to make his guacamole at every opportunity. It takes a little more time, but it is better than mine (shhh . . . don't tell my husband I just admitted that).

Ingredients

3 ripe Haas avocados, mashed

1 ripe plum tomato, diced

¼ yellow or red onion, chopped

½ jalapeno pepper, seeds removed, finely diced (more to taste if you like)

1 lime, juiced

1 handful cilantro, stems cut off, roughly chopped

½ teaspoon cumin

½ teaspoon garlic powder

¼ teaspoon onion powder

¼ teaspoon salt (more or less to taste)

⅛ teaspoon cayenne pepper, optional

Steps

Put the avocados, tomato, onion, jalapeno, lime juice, cilantro, cumin, garlic powder, onion powder, salt, and cayenne pepper into a bowl or a container with a tight-fitting lid. Mix until well combined. Cover tightly with a piece of plastic wrap pressed onto the guac to make sure no air gets in, and cover with the lid until ready to serve to keep the guacamole from turning brown. Store any leftovers in the fridge for one to two days (though it is unlikely that there will be leftovers) with the plastic wrap tightly covering the guacamole.

Desserts

Aunt Jann's Chocolate Chip Cookies
Makes about 4-5 dozen • Takes 45-60 minutes

Know which cookies are soft without emulsifiers? The kind right out of the oven. And cookies are actually pretty easy to make. Even if they don't come out perfectly, there's no such thing as a bad cookie. These cookies come courtesy of Aunt Jann (giving credit to Toll House for her inspiration) who is famous in our family for her cookies. And rightly so! Jann encourages the use of one bowl by starting with the wet ingredients, making for easier cleanup (Jann is the best!). Become famous in your family. Because this recipe makes so many cookies, your neighbors will like you more, too.

Ingredients
1 cup (2 sticks) salted butter, softened (see notes)
¾ cup granulated sugar
¾ cup (packed) light brown sugar
2 large eggs at room temperature, beaten
1 teaspoon vanilla extract
1 teaspoon baking soda
2¼ cups all-purpose flour
2 cups semisweet or dark chocolate chips, or a blend (see notes)

Steps
1. Preheat the oven to 375°F.
2. In a large mixing bowl or the bowl of a stand mixer, beat the butter and sugars on medium-high speed until light and fluffy.
3. Scrape down the sides of the bowl. Add the eggs and vanilla, and beat until well incorporated.
4. Add the baking soda and then slowly add the flour to the mixture a ½ cup at a time, making sure the flour is well mixed with each addition. Scrape down the sides of the bowl as needed.

5. Stir in the chocolate chips. If you want thicker, chewier cookies, pop the dough into the refrigerator for about an hour before baking. If you don't want to wait and don't mind thinner cookies, you can bake them right away.
6. Drop walnut-sized pieces of dough onto a cookie sheet, leaving 2 inches between cookies.
7. Bake one sheet at a time for 8–9 minutes or until the edges start to brown.
8. Transfer to a rack to cool.

Notes: If you have unsalted butter, add ½ teaspoon salt in step 4. Look for chocolate chips without lecithin in the ingredient list. If you can't find them, you can always purchase additive-free chocolate bars (which may be easier to come by) and chop the chocolate on your own. But don't sweat it: using chocolate chips with lecithin in homemade cookies still beats eating shelf-soft premade cookies!

Ridiculously Rich Chocolate Chunk Brownies
Makes 15–20 brownies • Takes 40 minutes

The good news is these brownies take about 40 minutes to throw together and bake. The bad news is these brownies are not for every day. They are strictly a special treat. You need a lot of butter and sugar to make them. They walk that fine line between brownies and fudge. And they are so good that they are gone in my house almost as fast as they are baked. So basically, proceed with caution.

Ingredients
1¾ cups sugar
1 cup (2 sticks) butter, melted and cooled
4 large eggs
2 teaspoons vanilla
⅔ cup cocoa powder
1 cup all-purpose flour
½ teaspoon salt
½ teaspoon baking powder
1 cup chocolate chunks or chips (see note above)

Steps

1. Preheat the oven to 350°F. Grease and flour a 9 × 13–inch baking dish.
2. Whisk together the sugar, butter, eggs, and vanilla in a large bowl.
3. Add the cocoa and whisk until well blended. Then add the flour, salt, and baking powder, and gently mix until fully incorporated.
4. Fold in the chocolate chunks.
5. Pour the batter into the prepared baking dish and spread to evenly distribute.
6. Bake for 26–29 minutes or until a toothpick inserted in the center comes out mostly clean—completely clean means you've overdone it. Let the brownies cool in the pan before cutting.

Olive Oil Cake

Adapted with the author's permission
from *A Family Farm in Tuscany* by Sarah Fioroni
Serves 10–12 • Takes 50 minutes

Now for something a little lighter. One of the best meals I've ever had was at a farm in Tuscany called Fattoria Poggio Alloro, run by Sarah Fioroni and her family. Our gaze rested on the verdant hills and freshly maintained fields as we were served course after course of farm-to-table dishes on wooden tables under the Tuscan sun. At the end of the meal, my husband disappeared to the small shop and later surprised me with Sarah's cookbook. As expected, everything we've made from it is delicious. This cake has become a staple in our home and is pretty much Sarah's recipe (I take full responsibility for the chocolate chips, which you can leave out if you want to stay true to her recipe). She brilliantly uses one container to measure everything. I use a dry ½-cup measuring cup for the measurements below.

Ingredients

1½ cups granulated sugar
4 large eggs

½ cup plain yogurt (Greek yogurt works very well)

2 cups all-purpose flour

½ cup extra-virgin olive oil

1 tablespoon baking powder

½ cup semisweet chocolate chips or mini chips, optional (see note on page 231)

Steps

1. Preheat the oven to 350°F. Thoroughly butter and flour a Bundt pan.
2. In a mixing bowl, cream the sugar and eggs with an electric mixer until light and fluffy. Add half of the yogurt and mix until well blended, then add the other half and mix again.
3. Add the flour to the mixture a ½ cup at a time, making sure the flour is well mixed with each addition. Scrape down the sides of the bowl as needed.
4. Add the olive oil and baking powder, and mix another 2–3 minutes, scraping down the sides at least once.
5. Gently fold the chocolate chips into the prepared batter if you're using them.
6. Pour the batter into the prepared Bundt pan.
7. Bake for 37–42 minutes or until a toothpick inserted in the center of the cake comes out clean. Cool in the pan for about 10 minutes, then run a knife along the sides to loosen the cake. Cover the pan with a wire rack and turn over, allowing the cake to slide onto the rack. Allow it to finish cooling on the rack.

Real Hot Cocoa

Serves 2 • Takes 5 minutes

Hot cocoa in packets is convenient and was a family favorite. So imagine my dismay when I discovered there were more additives than actual real-food ingredients on the label of our favorite hot chocolate drink. Luckily, I soon learned that making hot cocoa can be ridiculously easy. Many recipes will tell you to boil milk gently in a pot and whisk in the other ingredients when it comes to a boil. The problem with this is then you have a pot with yucky milk solids to scrape off and clean (I think this is why the packets were invented in the first place). Instead, I make it easy by microwaving my milk in a large Pyrex measuring cup, though any large microwave-safe glass container will do. It's not much harder than tearing open a packet.

Ingredients

2 cups milk (or your favorite additive-free milk substitute)
2 tablespoons cocoa powder
1–2 tablespoons granulated sugar depending on how sweet you like it

Steps

1. Microwave the milk for 2 minutes and 30 seconds on high.
2. Place half the cocoa powder and half the sugar into each mug.
3. Pour an ounce or two of milk into the mugs and whisk with a small whisk or fork until dissolved. Then add the rest of the milk and anything else you might like.

Note: You may get a few small clumps of cocoa but I think these are fine. If they bother you, they can be avoided by sifting the cocoa powder first.

Really Easy Homemade Whipped Cream
Serves 1-4 (depending on your love of
whipped cream) • Takes 2 minutes with a stand mixer

After making fresh whipped cream at home, I'm not sure I would buy the kind in a can again, even if I didn't suffer from IBS. This is just better and so easy. As noted in chapter 5, truly additive-free cream can be hard to find, but it's out there (one ingredient on the label is best). If you can't find it, well, DIY means fewer additives than the stuff in the can, which is a step in the right direction! The only downside to fresh whipped cream is that a container of real cream will only last a week or so after being opened. That's okay in my house. We make the sacrifice of devouring the whole thing in a few days. We do what we must.

This recipe uses a stand mixer. If you don't have one, a hand mixer works but may take a bit longer. If you don't have any mixer at all, you can whip up heavy cream with a whisk by hand. This will take you a few minutes more (and by minutes, I mean forever). But if you want an arm workout, go for it.

Ingredients

½ cup heavy or whipping cream

1 teaspoon to 1 tablespoon of granulated sugar (depending on how sweet you
   like it)

Steps

In the bowl of a stand mixer equipped with the whisk attachment, mix the cream and sugar on high speed for a minute or so. Watch it carefully and turn it off when you see the cream getting thick—you don't want to make butter.

Acknowledgments

I am forever grateful to the people who made this book possible.

To the people who nurtured and encouraged my writing: From my very first editor, Yves Colon at *The Miami Herald*, who believed in me at a time in my life when I needed that more than you could have known; to my mind-blowingly amazing editor, Claire Schulz at BenBella—you somehow figured out how to organize my thoughts and kept me on track. This book wouldn't be here without you. To Vy Tran, the person who would have been known as the designated pinch hitter in my residency, thank you for picking up the ball and getting it to the finish line (I know I completely mixed up sports metaphors here—sorry, Michael and Claire, who is probably dying to fix this). A special thanks to my copy editor, Ruth Strother . . . who, err, whom . . . I made suffer way more than any person should. And thanks to the entire team at BenBella, who was always there to answer my questions and worked so tirelessly to bring this book into the world. Thank you to my agent, Stacey Glick, for your guidance and for being there throughout the entire process. Thank you also to Andrea Guevara for championing my message and helping me stay on it!

To my friends who gave so freely of their time and energy: I want to send a special thank you to Jamie for being a sounding board and never-ending source of good advice. Thank you to Sandi for being generous beyond belief with your time and counsel. Thank you to the Wine and Words Book Club for always supporting me, especially Nova, Friederike, and the amazing Esther, who gave me so much thoughtful feedback. Hugs and love to Nieves and Caroline who led me to believe that I could do anything and listened to all my crazy ideas (also thanks for going through about one hundred versions of the subtitle with me). Thanks

Acknowledgments

to Meenakshi, who wouldn't let me leave Boston without cooking lessons and a trip to the Indian grocery store—you helped get me started making food I didn't think I could at first. Thank you, Allison, for your endless positivity and insights into the inner workings of a commercial kitchen. To Natasha, thanks for being an early cheerleader (but only in the metaphorical sense!) and for introducing me to the phenomenal Yalda Alaoui, who is an inspiration. A giant thank you to Pramita for always being there to listen for more than twenty years and for sharing your stories with me, too. *Obrigada* to Kelly at Mission—you never say *no* or *can't* and are an absolute force of nature.

To the people who made sure my medical information was accurate and understandable (if errors or oversights were made, they are mine): Thank you to Drs. Carlos Monteiro and Benoit Chassaing for your patience and generosity and for forgiving me for my nonexistent abilities in Portuguese and French. Thank you to Professor Barbara Olendzki, who made sure I didn't forget how important real prebiotics are! Thank you also to Dr. Sarah Steinberg, Sara Baer-Sinnott, and Marit Kolby Zinöcker, for being so generous with your time and ideas. A special thank you to my beta readers, Drs. Peter Lio, Julie Servoss, and Elliot Ellis, for your encouragement and for keeping it EBM-focused.

And finally, thank you to my husband, Michael, for supporting me in all my endeavors and for making our lives a delicious adventure.

Notes

Chapter 1: The Microbiome and the
Rise of Diet-Related Diseases

1   P. Weintraub, "The Doctor Who Drank Infectious Broth, Gave Himself an Ulcer, and Solved a Medical Mystery," *Discover Magazine*, April 8, 2010, accessed August 10, 2022, https://www.discovermagazine.com/health/the-doctor-who-drank-infectious-broth-gave-himself-an-ulcer-and-solved-a-medical-mystery.

2   A. Almeida, A. L. Mitchell, M. Boland, et al., "A New Genomic Blueprint of the Human Gut Microbiota," *Nature* 568 (2019): 499–504, doi:10.1038/s41586-019-0965-1.

3   J. K. Vanamala, R. Knight, T. D. Spector, "Can Your Microbiome Tell You What to Eat?," *Cell Metab*, 22, no. 6 (2015): 960–961, doi:10.1016/j.cmet.2015.11.009.

4   B. O. Schroeder, "Fight Them or Feed Them: How the Intestinal Mucus Layer Manages the Gut Microbiota," *Gastroenterol Rep* (Oxf), 7, no. 1 (2019): 3–12, doi:10.1093/gastro/goy052.

5   P. G. Farup, K. Rudi, K. Hestad, "Faecal Short-Chain Fatty Acids—a Diagnostic Biomarker for Irritable Bowel Syndrome?," *BMC Gastroenterol*, 16 no. 1 (2016): 51, doi:10.1186/s12876-016-0446-z.

6   A. Leshem, E. Segal, E. Elinav, "The Gut Microbiome and Individual-Specific Responses to Diet," *mSystems*, 5 no. 5 (2020): e00665—20, doi:10.1128/mSystems.00665-20.

7   American Diabetes Association, "Statistics About Diabetes," accessed January 17, 2022, https://www.diabetes.org/resources/statistics/statistics-about-diabetes.

8   CDC's Division of Diabetes Translation, "Long-term Trends in Diabetes," April 2017, accessed January 17, 2022, https://www.cdc.gov/diabetes/statistics/slides/long_term_trends.pdf.

9   F. Rauber, M. L. da Costa Louzada, E. M. Steele, et al., "Ultra-Processed Food Consumption and Chronic Non-Communicable Diseases-Related Dietary Nutrient Profile in the UK (2008–2014)," *Nutrients*, 10 no. 5 (2018): 587, doi:10.3390/nu10050587; Obesity Society, "U.S. Adult Consumption of Added Sugars Increased by More Than 30 Percent Over Three Decades," *ScienceDaily*, November 4, 2014, accessed May 29, 2022, www.sciencedaily.com/releases/2014/11/141104141731.htm.

10 S. Basu, P. Yoffe, N. Hills, et al., "The Relationship of Sugar to Population-Level Diabetes Prevalence: An Econometric Analysis of Repeated Cross-Sectional Data," *PLoS One*, 8 no. 2 (2013): e57873, doi:10.1371/journal.pone.0057873.

11 H. Gardener, Y. P. Moon, T. Rundek, et al., "Diet Soda and Sugar-Sweetened Soda Consumption in Relation to Incident Diabetes in the Northern Manhattan Study," *Curr Dev Nutr*, 2 no. 5 (2018): nzy008, doi:10.1093/cdn/nzy008.

12 F. J. Ruiz-Ojed, J. Plaza-Díaz, M. J. Sáez-Lara, et al., "Effects of Sweeteners on the Gut Microbiota: A Review of Experimental Studies and Clinical Trials, *Adv Nutr*, 10 suppl. 1 (2019): S31–S48, doi:10.1093/advances/nmy037, [published correction appears in *Adv Nutr.*, 11 no 2 (March 2020): 468].

13 D. Partridge, K. A. Lloyd, J. M. Rhodes, et al., "Food Additives: Assessing the Impact of Exposure to Permitted Emulsifiers on Bowel and Metabolic Health—Introducing the FADiets Study," *Nutr Bull*, 44 no. 4 (2019): 329–349, doi:10.1111/nbu.12408.

14 M. Gurung, Z. Li, H. You, et al., "Role of Gut Microbiota in Type 2 Diabetes Pathophysiology," *EBioMedicine*, 51 (2020):102590, doi:10.1016/j.ebiom.2019.11.051.

15 Gurung, et al., "Roll of Gut."

16 G. M. Reaven, "Syndrome X: A Short History," *Ochsner Journal*, 3 no. 3 (July 2001):124–125.

17 M. Aguilar, T. Bhuket, S. Torres, et al., "Prevalence of the Metabolic Syndrome in the United States, 2003–2012," *JAMA*, 313 no. 19 (2015):1973–1974, doi:10.1001/jama.2015.4260.

18 K. Dabke, G. Hendrick, S. Devkota, "The Gut Microbiome and Metabolic Syndrome," *J Clin Invest*, 129 no. 10 (2019): 4050–4057, doi:10.1172/JCI129194.

19 B. Chassaing, O. Koren, J. K. Goodrich, et al., "Dietary Emulsifiers Impact the Mouse Gut Microbiota Promoting Colitis and Metabolic Syndrome, *Nature*, 519 no. 7541 (2015): 92–96, doi:10.1038/nature14232, [published correction appears in *Nature*, 536 no. 7615 (Aug 11, 2016): 238].

20 Z. Jiang, M. Zhao, H. Zhang, et al., "Antimicrobial Emulsifier-Glycerol Monolaurate Induces Metabolic Syndrome, Gut Microbiota Dysbiosis, and Systemic Low-Grade Inflammation in Low-Fat Diet Fed Mice," *Mol Nutr Food Res*, 62 no. 3 (2018), doi:10.1002/mnfr.201700547.

21 B. Chassaing, C. Compher, B. Bonhomme, et. al., "Randomized Controlled-Feeding Study of Dietary Emulsifier Carboxymethylcellulose Reveals Detrimental Impacts on the Gut Microbiota and Metabolome," *Gastroenterology*, 162 no. 3, (2022): 743–756, doi:10.1053/j.gastro.2021.11.006.

22 C. C. Lindenmeyer, A. J. McCullough, "The Natural History of Nonalcoholic Fatty Liver Disease—An Evolving View," *Clin Liver Dis*, 22 no. 1 (2018): 11–21, doi:10.1016/j.cld.2017.08.003.

23 I. Pierantonelli, G. Svegliati-Baroni, "Nonalcoholic Fatty Liver Disease: Basic Pathogenetic Mechanisms in the Progression from NAFLD to NASH," *Transplantation*, 103 no. 1 (2019): e1–e13, doi:10.1097/TP.0000000000002480.

24 J. Ludwig, T. R. Viggiano, D. B. McGill, et al., "Nonalcoholic Steatohepatitis: Mayo Clinic Experiences with a Hitherto Unnamed Disease," *Mayo Clin Proc* 55 no. 7 (1980): 434–438.

25 B. Li, C. Zhang, Y. T. Zhan, "Nonalcoholic Fatty Liver Disease Cirrhosis: A Review of Its Epidemiology, Risk Factors, Clinical Presentation, Diagnosis, Management, and Prognosis," *Can J Gastroenterol Hepatol*, 2018 (July 2, 2018): 2784537, doi:10.1155/2018/2784537.

26 F. Nassir, R. S. Rector, G. M. Hammoud, et al., "Pathogenesis and Prevention of Hepatic Steatosis," *Gastroenterol Hepatol* (N Y), 11 no.3 (2015): 167–175.

27 M. V. Salguero, M. A. I. Al-Obaide, R. Singh, et al., "Dysbiosis of Gram-Negative Gut Microbiota and the Associated Serum Lipopolysaccharide Exacerbates Inflammation in Type 2 Diabetic Patients with Chronic Kidney Disease," *Exp Ther Med*, 18 no. 5 (2019): 3461–3469. doi:10.3892/etm.2019.7943.

28 R. Loomba, V. Seguritan, W. Li, et al., "Gut Microbiome-Based Metagenomic Signature for Non-Invasive Detection of Advanced Fibrosis in Human Nonalcoholic Fatty Liver Disease," *Cell Metab*, 25 no.5 (2017): 1054–1062.e5, doi:10.1016/j.cmet.2017.04.001, [published correction appears in *Cell Metab*, 30 no. 3 (Sep. 3, 2019): 607].

29 J. W. Park, S. E. Kim, N. Y. Lee, et al., "Role of Microbiota-Derived Metabolites in Alcoholic and Non-Alcoholic Fatty Liver Diseases," *Int J Mol Sci*, 23 no. 1 (Dec. 31, 2021): 426, doi:10.3390/ijms23010426.

30 "Inflammatory Bowel Disease (IBD)," Centers for Disease Control and Prevention, accessed January 19, 2022, https://www.cdc.gov/ibd/data-statistics.htm.

31 "Collagenous and Lymphocytic Colitis," Johns Hopkins Medicine, accessed January 19, 2022, https://www.hopkinsmedicine.org/gastroenterology_hepatology/_pdfs/small_large_intestine/collagenous_lymphocytic_colitis.pdf.

32 Georgia State News Hub, "Ubiquitous Food Additive Alters Human Microbiota and Intestinal Environment," Georgia State University, November 30, 2021, accessed May 29, 2022, https://news.gsu.edu/2021/11/30/ubiquitous-food-additive-alters-human-microbiota-and-intestinal-environment/.

33 C. L. Roberts, S. L. Rushworth, E. Richman, et al., "Hypothesis: Increased Consumption of Emulsifiers as an Explanation for the Rising Incidence of Crohn's Disease," *J Crohns Colitis*, 7 no. 4 (2013): 338–341, doi:10.1016/j.crohns.2013.01.004.

34 B. E. Lacy, N. K. Patel, "Rome Criteria and a Diagnostic Approach to Irritable Bowel Syndrome," *J Clin Med*, 6 no. 11 (Oct. 26, 2017): 99, doi:10.3390/jcm6110099.

35 C. Canavan, J. West, T. Card, "The Epidemiology of Irritable Bowel Syndrome, *Clin Epidemiol*, 6 (Feb. 4, 2014): 71–80, doi: 10.2147/CLEP.S40245.

36 O. S. Palsson, J. S. Baggish, M. J. Turner, et al., "IBS Patients Show Frequent Fluctuations Between Loose/Watery and Hard/Lumpy Stools: Implications for Treatment," *Am J Gastroenterol*, 107 no. 2 (2012): 286–295, doi:10.1038/ajg.2011.358.

37 E. J. Krajicek, S. L. Hansel, "Small Intestinal Bacterial Overgrowth: A Primary Care Review," *Mayo Clin Proc*, 91 no. 12 (2016): 1828–1833, doi:10.1016/j.mayocp.2016.07.025.

38 M. Pimentel, "Evaluating a Bacterial Hypothesis in IBS Using a Modification of Koch's Postulates: Part 1," *Am J Gastroentero*, 105 no. 4 (Apr. 2010): 718–21, doi: 10.1038/ajg.2009.678.

39 H. C. Lin, "Small Intestinal Bacterial Overgrowth: A Framework for Understanding Irritable Bowel Syndrome," *JAMA*, 292 no. 7 (2004): 852–858. doi: https://doi.org/10.1001/jama.292.7.852.

Notes

40   M. Pimentel, E. J. Chow, H. C. Lin, "Eradication of Small Intestinal Bacterial Overgrowth Reduces Symptoms of Irritable Bowel Syndrome," *Am J Gastroenterol*, 95 no. 12 (2000): 3503–3506, doi:10.1111/j.1572-0241.2000.03368.x.

41   C. J. Black, A. C. Ford, "How Effective Are Antibiotics for the Treatment of Irritable Bowel Syndrome," *Expert Opin Pharmacother*, 21 no. 18 (2020): 2195–2197, doi:10.1080/146565 66.2020.1808623.

42   D. Ternes, J. Karta, M. Tsenkova, et al., "Microbiome in Colorectal Cancer: How to Get from Meta-omics to Mechanism?," *Trends Microbiol*, 28 no. 5 (2020): 401–423, doi:10.1016/ j.tim.2020.01.001. [published correction appears in *Trends Microbiol*, 28 no. 8 (Aug. 2020): 698].

43   J. M. Rhodes, "The Role of *Escherichia coli* in Inflammatory Bowel Disease," *Gut*, 56 no. 5 (2007): 610–612, doi:10.1136/gut.2006.111872.

44   T. Christofi, S. Panayidou, I. Dieronitou, et al., "Metabolic Output Defines *Escherichia coli* as a Health-Promoting Microbe Against Intestinal *Pseudomonas aeruginosa*," *Sci Rep*, 9 no. 1 (Oct. 8, 2019): 14463, doi:10.1038/s41598-019-51058-3.

45   E. Rinninella, P. Raoul, M. Cintoni, et al., "What Is the Healthy Gut Microbiota Composition? A Changing Ecosystem across Age, Environment, Diet, and Diseases," *Microorganisms*, 7 no. 1 (Jan. 10, 2019): 14, doi:10.3390/microorganisms7010014.

46   "About the Young-Onset Colorectal Cancer Center," Dana Farber Cancer Institute Young-Onset Colorectal Cancer Center, accessed January 20, 2022, https://www.dana-farber.org/ young-onset-colorectal-cancer-center/.

47   T. Fiolet, B. Srour, L. Sellem, et al., "Consumption of Ultra-Processed Foods and Cancer Risk: Results from NutriNet-Santé Prospective Cohort," *BMJ*, 360 (Feb. 14, 2018): k322, doi:10.1136/bmj.k322.

48   E. Viennois, B. Chassaing, "Consumption of Select Dietary Emulsifiers Exacerbates the Development of Spontaneous Intestinal Adenoma," *Int J Mol Sci.*, 22 no. 5 (March 5, 2021): 2602, doi:10.3390/ijms22052602.

49   S. R. Cox, J. O. Lindsay, S. Fromentin, et al., "Effects of Low FODMAP Diet on Symptoms, Fecal Microbiome, and Markers of Inflammation in Patients with Quiescent Inflammatory Bowel Disease in a Randomized Trial," *Gastroenterology*, 158 no. 1 (2020): 176–188.e7, doi:10.1053/j.gastro.2019.09.024; Y. Jiang, K. Jarr, C. Layton, et al., "Therapeutic Implications of Diet in Inflammatory Bowel Disease and Related Immune-Mediated Inflammatory Diseases," *Nutrients*, 13 no. 3 (Mar 10, 2021): 890, doi:10.3390/nu13030890.

50   A. Lenhart, W. D. Chey, "A Systematic Review of the Effects of Polyols on Gastrointestinal Health and Irritable Bowel Syndrome," *Adv Nutr*, 8 no. 4 (Jul 6, 2017): 587–596, doi: 10.3945/an.117.015560.

51   L. A. Bazzano, J. He, L. G. Ogden, et al., "Legume Consumption and Risk of Coronary Heart Disease in US Men and Women: NHANES I Epidemiologic Follow-Up Study," *Arch Intern Med*, 161 no. 21 (2001): 2573–2578, doi:10.1001/archinte.161.21.2573.

52   J. Molina-Infante, J. SerraJ, F. Fernandez-Bañares, et al., "The Low-FODMAP Diet for Irritable Bowel Syndrome: Lights and Shadows," *Gastroenterol Hepatol*, 39 no. 2 (2016): 55–65, doi:10.1016/j.gastrohep.2015.07.009.

53 G. Riccardi, A. A. Rivellese, "Effects of Dietary Fiber and Carbohydrate on Glucose and Lipoprotein Metabolism in Diabetic Patients," *Diabetes Care*, 14 no. 12 (1991): 1115–1125, doi:10.2337/diacare.14.12.1115.

54 E. Altobelli, V. Del Negro, P.M. Angeletti, et al., "Low-FODMAP Diet Improves Irritable Bowel Syndrome Symptoms: A Meta-Analysis," *Nutrients*, 9 no. 9 (Aug. 26, 2017): 940, doi: 10.3390/nu9090940; J. Dionne, A. C. Ford, Y. Yuan, et al., "A Systematic Review and Meta-Analysis Evaluating the Efficacy of a Gluten-Free Diet and a Low FODMAPs Diet in Treating Symptoms of Irritable Bowel Syndrome," *Am J Gastroenterol*, 113 no. 9 (2018):1290–1300, doi: 10.1038/s41395-018-0195-4.

55 V. K. Gupta, K. Y. Cunningham, B. Hur, et al., "Gut Microbial Determinants of Clinically Important Improvement in Patients with Rheumatoid Arthritis," *Genome Med*, 13 no. 1 (Sep. 14, 2021): 149, doi:10.1186/s13073-021-00957-0.

56 M. Valles-Colomer, G. Falony, Y. Darzi, et al., "The Neuroactive Potential of the Human Gut Microbiota in Quality of Life and Depression," *Nat Microbiol*, 4 no. 4 (2019): 623–632, doi:10.1038/s41564-018-0337-x.

57 E. Sanchez-Rodriguez, A. Egea-Zorrilla, J. Plaza-Díaz, et al., "The Gut Microbiota and Its Implication in the Development of Atherosclerosis and Related Cardiovascular Diseases," *Nutrients*, 12 no. 3 (Feb 26, 2020): 605, doi:10.3390/nu12030605.

58 K. W. Della Corte, I. Perrar, K. J. Penczynski, et al., "Effect of Dietary Sugar Intake on Biomarkers of Subclinical Inflammation: A Systematic Review and Meta-Analysis of Intervention Studies," *Nutrients*, 10 no. 5 (May 12, 2018): 606, doi:10.3390/nu10050606.

59 J. Jin, J. Li, Y. Gan, et al., "Red Meat Intake is Associated with Early Onset of Rheumatoid Arthritis: A Cross-Sectional Study," *Sci Rep*, 11 no. 1 (Mar 11, 2021): 5681, doi:10.1038/s41598-021-85035-6.

60 N. Narula, E. C. L. Wong, M. Dehghan, et al., "Association of Ultra-processed Food Intake with Risk of Inflammatory Bowel Disease: Prospective Cohort Study," *BMJ*, 374 (Jul 14, 2021): n1554, doi:10.1136/bmj.n1554; K. H. Allin , R. C. Ungaro, M. Agrawal, "Ultraprocessed Foods and the Risk of Inflammatory Bowel Disease: Is It Time to Modify Diet?," *Gastroenterology*, 162 no. 2 (2022): 652–654, doi:10.1053/j.gastro.2021.09.053.

61 S. Deleu, K. Machiels, J. Raes, et al., "Short Chain Fatty Acids and Its Producing Organisms: An Overlooked Therapy for IBD?," *EBioMedicine*, 66 (2021): 103293, doi:10.1016/j.ebiom.2021.103293.

62 B. van der Hee, J. M. Wells, "Microbial Regulation of Host Physiology by Short-Chain Fatty Acids," *Trends Microbiol*, 29 no. 8 (2021): 700–712, doi:10.1016/j.tim.2021.02.001.

63 M. Luu, Z. Riester, A. Baldrich, et al., "Microbial Short-Chain Fatty Acids Modulate CD8+ T Cell Responses and Improve Adoptive Immunotherapy for Cancer," *Nat Commun*, 12 no. 1 (Jul 1, 2021): 4077, doi:10.1038/s41467-021-24331-1.

64 L. Sköldstam, L. Hagfors, G. Johansson, "An Experimental Study of a Mediterranean Diet Intervention for Patients with Rheumatoid Arthritis," *Ann Rheum Dis*, 62 no. 3 (2003): 208–214, doi:10.1136/ard.62.3.208; S. P. Juraschek, L. C. Kovell, L. J. Appel, et al., "Effects of Diet and Sodium Reduction on Cardiac Injury, Strain, and Inflammation: The DASH-Sodium Trial," *J Am Coll Cardiol*, 77 no. 21 (2021): 2625–2634, doi:10.1016/j.jacc.2021.03.320.

65 F. Juul, N. Parekh, E. Martinez-Steele, et al., "Ultra-Processed Food Consumption Among US Adults from 2001 to 2018," *Am J Clin Nutr*, 115 no. 1 (2022): 211–221, doi:10.1093/ajcn/nqab305; L. Wang, E. Martínez Steele, M. Du, et al., "Trends in Consumption of Ultraprocessed Foods Among US Youths Aged 2–19 Years, 1999–2018," *JAMA*, 326 no. 6 (2021): 519–530, doi:10.1001/jama.2021.10238.

66 NCI Staff, "Why Is Colorectal Cancer Rising Rapidly Among Young Adults?," *Cancer Currents* (blog), National Cancer Institute, November 5, 2020, accessed January 14, 2022, https://www.cancer.gov/news-events/cancer-currents-blog/2020/colorectal-cancer-rising-younger-adults.

Chapter 2: What's Gone Wrong with Our Food?

67 C. Reinoso Webb, I. Koboziev, K. L. Furr, et al., "Protective and Pro-Inflammatory Roles of Intestinal Bacteria," *Pathophysiology*, 23 no. 2 (2016): 67–80, doi:10.1016/j.pathophys.2016.02.002; E. Viennois, A. Bretin, P. E. Dubé, et al., "Dietary Emulsifiers Directly Impact Adherent-Invasive *E. coli* Gene Expression to Drive Chronic Intestinal Inflammation," *Cell Rep*, 33 no. 1 (2020): 108229, doi:10.1016/j.celrep.2020.108229; A. Levine, R. Sigall Boneh, E. Wine, "Evolving Role of Diet in the Pathogenesis and Treatment of Inflammatory Bowel Diseases," *Gut*, 67 no. 9 (2018): 1726–1738, doi:10.1136/gutjnl-2017-315866.

68 Carlos Monteiro, "E24: Carlos Monteiro on the Dangers of Ultra-Processed Foods," Duke Sanford World Food Policy Center, March 26, 2019, podcast, https://wfpc.sanford.duke.edu/podcasts/carlos-monteiro-dangers-ultra-processed-foods/.

69 BBC News, "Chorleywood: The Bread That Changed Britain," June 7, 2011, accessed March 10, 2022, www.bbc.com/news/magazine-13670278.

70 D. Pszczola, "Plot Thickens, as Gums Add Special Effects.," *Food Technology Magazine*, December 1, 2003, accessed June 26, 2020, https://www.ift.org/news-and-publications/food-technology%20magazine/%20issues/2003/december/columns/ingredients.

71 B. Wilson, *The Way We Eat Now: How the Food Revolution Has Transformed Our Lives, Our Bodies, and Our World* (New York: Basic Books, 2019).

72 M. K. Zinöcker, I. A. Lindseth, "The Western Diet-Microbiome-Host Interaction and Its Role in Metabolic Disease," *Nutrients*, 10 no. 3 (Mar 17, 2018): 365, doi:10.3390/nu10030365.

73 Ministry of Health of Brazil, "Dietary Guidelines for the Brazilian Population, Secretariat of Health Care Primary Health Care Department, 2015, accessed September 16, 2021, http://bvsms.saude.gov.br/bvs/publicacoes/dietary_guidelines_brazilian_population.pdf.

74 Carlos A. Monteiro, in discussion with the author, September 2021.

75 US Food and Drug Administration, "Food Ingredient and Packaging Terms," current as of January 4, 2018, accessed April 21, 2020, https://www.fda.gov/food/food-ingredients-packaging/food-ingredient-packaging-terms.

76 Food and Safety Authority of Ireland, "Introduction," last reviewed April 8, 2021, accessed August 26, 2021, https://www.fsai.ie/legislation/food_legislation/food_additives/introduction.html.

77   M. Pollan, *In Defense of Food: An Eater's Manifesto* (New York: Penguin Press, 2008), 51–54.

78   T. G. Neltner, H. M. Alger, J. E. Leonard, et al., "Data Gaps in Toxicity Testing of Chemicals Allowed in Food in the United States," *Reprod Toxicol*, 42 (2013): 85–94, doi:10.1016/j.reprotox.2013.07.023.

79   Neltner, et al., "Data Gaps," 2013.

80   D. Partridge, K. A. Lloyd, J. M. Rhodes, et al., "Food Additives: Assessing the Impact of Exposure to Permitted Emulsifiers on Bowel and Metabolic Health: Introducing the FADiets Study," *Nutr Bull.*, 44 no. 4 (2019): 329–349, doi:10.1111/nbu.12408.

81   Partridge, et al., "Food Additives," 2019.

82   S. Naimi, E. Viennois, A. T. Gewirtz, et al., "Direct Impact of Commonly Used Dietary Emulsifiers on Human Gut Microbiota," *Microbiome*, 9 no. 1 (Mar 22, 2021): 66, doi:10.1186/s40168-020-00996-6.

83   Benoit Chassaing, in discussion with the author, September 2021.

84   J. Adams, K. Hofman, J. C. Moubarac, et al., "Public Health Response to Ultra-Processed Food and Drinks," *BMJ*, 369 (Jun 26, 2020): m2391, doi:10.1136/bmj.m2391.

85   M. Champ, "Resistant Starch," in *Starch in Food Structure, Function and Applications*, ed. A-C. Eliasson (Cambridge, England: Woodhead Publishing Limited, 2004), 560–574.

86   M. Younes, P. Aggett, F. Aguilar, et al., "Re-Evaluation of Celluloses E 460(i), E 460 (ii), E 461, E 462, E 463, E 464, E 465, E 466, E 468, and E 469 as Food Additives," *EFSA Journal*, 16 no. 1 (Sep 27, 2018), doi: 10.2903/j.efsa.2018.5047.

87   Younes, et al., "Re-Evaluation of Celluloses," 2018.

88   Champ, "Resistant Starch," 2004.

89   J. R. Lupton, "Microbial Degradation Products Influence Colon Cancer Risk: The Butyrate Controversy," *J Nutr*, 134 no. 2 (Feb 2004): 479–482.

90   J. Slavin, "Fiber and Prebiotics: Mechanisms and Health Benefits," *Nutrients*, 5 no. 4 (Apr 22, 2013): 1417–1435, doi: 10.3390/nu5041417.

91   Y. S. Seo, H. B. Lee, Y. Kim, et al., "Dietary Carbohydrate Constituents Related to Gut Dysbiosis and Health," *Microorganisms*, 8 no. 3 (Mar 18, 2020): 427, doi:10.3390/microorganisms8030427.

92   F. Juul, et al., "Ultra-Processed Food Consumption," 2022.

93   W. Stremmel, A. Hanemann, R. Ehehalt, et al., "Phosphatidylcholine (Lecithin) and the Mucus Layer: Evidence of Therapeutic Efficacy in Ulcerative Colitis?," *Dig Dis*, 28 no. 3 (2010): 490–496, doi: 10.1159/000320407.

94   Y. Merga, B. J. Campbell, J. M. Rhodes, "Mucosal Barrier, Bacteria and Inflammatory Bowel Disease: Possibilities for Therapy," *Dig Dis*, 32 no. 4 (2014): 475–483, doi:10.1159/000358156.

95   "Lecithin," Health Encyclopedia, University of Rochester Medical Center, accessed December 18, 2019, https://www.urmc.rochester.edu/encyclopedia/content.aspx?contenttypeid=19&contentid=Lecithin.

96   Code of Federal Regulations, Title 21, US Food and Drug Administration, updated October 21, 2021, accessed January 15, 2022, https://www.accessdata.fda.gov/scripts/cdrh/cfdocs/cfcfr/CFRSearch.cfm?fr=184.1400&SearchTerm=lecithin.

97 S. David, C. Shani Levi, L. Fahoum, et al., "Revisiting the Carrageenan Controversy: Do We Really Understand the Digestive Fate and Safety of Carrageenan in Our Foods?," *Food Funct*, 9 no. 3 (2018): 1344–1352, doi:10.1039/c7fo01721a.

98 D. Charles, "USDA Defies Advisors, Allows Carrageenan to Keep Organic Label," The Salt: What's On Your Plate, NPR, April 14, 2018, accessed November 6, 2019, https://www.npr.org/sections/thesalt/2018/04/04/599550018/usda-sides-with-big-organic-to-allow-emulsifier-to-keep-organic-label.

99 EFSA Panel on Food Additives and Nutrient Sources added to Food (ANS), M. Younes, P. Aggett, et al., "Re-Evaluation of Carrageenan (E 407) and Processed Eucheuma Seaweed (E 407a) as Food Additives," *EFSA J*, 16 no. 4 (Apr 26, 2018): e05238, doi:10.2903/j.efsa.2018.5238.

100 Partridge, et al., "Food Additives," 2019.

101 J. V. Martino, J. Van Limbergen, L. E. Cahill, "The Role of Carrageenan and Carboxymethylcellulose in the Development of Intestinal Inflammation," *Front Pediatr*, 5 (May 1, 2017): 96, doi:10.3389/fped.2017.00096.

102 C. L. Roberts, A. V. Keita, S. H. Duncan, et al., "Translocation of Crohn's Disease *Escherichia coli* across M-Cells: Contrasting Effects of Soluble Plant Fibres and Emulsifiers," *Gut*, 59 no. 10 (2010): 1331–1339, doi:10.1136/gut.2009.195370.

103 A. Swidsinski, V. Ung, B. C. Sydora, et al., "Bacterial Overgrowth and Inflammation of Small Intestine After Carboxymethylcellulose Ingestion in Genetically Susceptible Mice," *Inflamm Bowel Dis*, 15 no. 3 (2009): 359–364, doi:10.1002/ibd.20763; F. Laudisi, D. Di Fusco, V. Dinallo, et al., "The Food Additive Maltodextrin Promotes Endoplasmic Reticulum Stress-Driven Mucus Depletion and Exacerbates Intestinal Inflammation," *Cell Mol Gastroenterol Hepatol*, 7 no. 2 (2019): 457–473, doi:10.1016/j.jcmgh.2018.09.002.

104 A. Levine, J. M. Rhodes, J. O. Lindsay, et al., "Dietary Guidance from the International Organization for the Study of Inflammatory Bowel Diseases," *Clin Gastroenterol Hepatol*, 18 no. 6 (2020): 1381–1392, doi:10.1016/j.cgh.2020.01.046.

105 H. Yanai, A. Levine, A. Hirsch, et al., "The Crohn's Disease Exclusion Diet for Induction and Maintenance of Remission in Adults with Mild-to-Moderate Crohn's Disease (CDED-AD): An Open-Label, Pilot, Randomised Trial," *Lancet Gastroenterol Hepatol*, 7 no. 1 (2022): 49–59, doi:10.1016/S2468-1253(21)00299-5.

106 Barbara Olendzki, in discussion with the author, September 2021.

Chapter 3: Why It's Hard to Eat Real Food

107 "Quick Facts: West Palm Beach City, Florida," United States Census Bureau, July 1, 2021, accessed January 15, 2022, www.census.gov/quickfacts/westpalmbeachcityflorida.

108 B. K. Cheon, Y. Y. Hong, "Mere Experience of Low Subjective Socioeconomic Status Stimulates Appetite and Food Intake," *Proc Natl Acad Sci U S A*, 114 no. 1 (2017): 72–77, doi:10.1073/pnas.1607330114.

109 E. Ruggiero, S. Esposito, S. Costanzo, et al., "Ultra-Processed Food Consumption and Its Correlates Among Italian Children, Adolescents and Adults from the Italian Nutrition & Health Survey (INHES) Cohort Study," *Public Health Nutr*, 24 no. 18 (Dec 2021): 6258–6271, doi:10.1017/S1368980021002767.

110 Andrade G. Calixto, C. Julia, V. Deschamps, et al., "Consumption of Ultra-Processed Food and Its Association with Sociodemographic Characteristics and Diet Quality in a Representative Sample of French Adults," *Nutrients*, 13 no. 2 (Feb 20, 2021): 682, doi:10.3390/nu13020682.

111 Partridge, et al., "Food Additives," 2019.

112 "Clean Eating: The Good and the Bad," Harvard Health Publishing Harvard Medical School, October 23, 2020, accessed March 10, 2022, https://www.health.harvard.edu/staying-healthy/clean-eating-the-good-and-the-bad.

113 M. Garber, "The Most Contentious Meal of the Day," *The Atlantic*, June 19, 2016, accessed August 31, 2020, https://www.theatlantic.com/entertainment/archive/2016/06/breakfast-the-most-contentious-meal-of-the-day/487220/.

114 D. Blum, *The Poison Squad* (New York: Penguin Press, 2018), 186–190.

115 M. A. Antje, A. Siepelmeyer, A. Holz, et al., "Effect of Consumption of Chicory Inulin on Bowel Function in Healthy Subjects with Constipation: A Randomized, Double-Blind, Placebo-Controlled Trial," *Int J Food Sci Nutr*, 68 no. 1 (2017): 82–89, doi:10.1080/09637486.2016.1212819.

116 M. S. Desai, A. M. Seekatz, N. M. Koropatkin, et al., "A Dietary Fiber-Deprived Gut Microbiota Degrades the Colonic Mucus Barrier and Enhances Pathogen Susceptibility," *Cell*, 167 no. 5 (2016): 1339–1353.e21, doi:10.1016/j.cell.2016.10.043.

117 V. Singh, B. S. Yeoh, B. Chassaing, et al., "Dysregulated Microbial Fermentation of Soluble Fiber Induces Cholestatic Liver Cancer," *Cell*, 175 no. 3 (2018): 679–694.e22, doi:10.1016/j.cell.2018.09.004.

118 A. M. Valdes, J. Walter, E. Segal, et al., "Role of the Gut Microbiota in Nutrition and Health," *BMJ*, 361 (Jun 13, 2018): k2179, doi:10.1136/bmj.k2179.

119 S. Wadyka, "Safety of Probiotic Supplements Is Not Guaranteed, Study Says," *Consumer Reports*, July 16, 2018, accessed October 23, 2019, https://www.consumerreports.org/dietary-supplements/safety-of-probiotic-supplements-is-not-guaranteed-study-says/.

120 H. C. Wastyk, G. K. Fragiadakis, D. Perelman, et al., "Gut-Microbiota-Targeted Diets Modulate Human Immune Status," *Cell*, 184 no. 16 (2021): 4137–4153.e14, doi:10.1016/j.cell.2021.06.019.

121 Zinöcker and Lindseth, "The Western Diet," 2018.

122 K. D. Brownell, J. L. Pomeranz, "The Trans-Fat Ban: Food Regulation and Long-Term Health," *N Engl J Med*, 370 no. 19 (May 8, 2014): 1773–1775, doi: 10.1056/NEJMp1314072.

123 L. Schnabel, C. Buscail, J. M. Sabate, et al., "Association Between Ultra-Processed Food Consumption and Functional Gastrointestinal Disorders: Results from the French NutriNet-Santé Cohort," *American Journal of Gastroenterology*, 113 no. 8 (Aug 2018): 1217–1228, doi: 10.1038/s41395-018-0137-1.

124 "Food Safety: Re-Evaluation," European Commission, accessed May 27, 2021, https://ec. europa.eu/food/safety/food_improvement_agents/additives/re-evaluation_en.

125 "Nearly Half the Experts from the European Food Safety Authority Have Financial Conflicts of Interest," Corporate Europe Observatory, June 14, 2017, accessed January 15, 2022, https:// corporateeurope.org/en/pressreleases/2017/06/nearly-half-experts-european-food-safety-authority-have-financial-conflicts.

126 M. Nestle, *Unsavory Truth: How Food Companies Skew the Science of What We Eat* (New York: Basic Books, 2018).

127 A. C. Lopez, "Adding Insult to Injury: Food Additives and US/EU International Trade," *Notre Dame Journal of International & Comparative Law*, 2016, http://scholarship.law.nd.edu/ndjicl/vol6/iss1/16.

128 T. Lang, E. P. Millstone "Post-Brexit Food Standards," *Lancet*, 393 no. 10177 (2019): 1199, doi:10.1016/S0140-6736(19)30540-9.

129 Nestle, *Unsavory Truth*, 2018.

130 A. H. Lichtenstein, L. J. Appel, M. Vadiveloo, et al., "2021 Dietary Guidance to Improve Cardiovascular Health: A Scientific Statement from the American Heart Association," *Circulation*, 144 (2021): e472–e487, doi:10.1161/CIR.0000000000001031.

131 S. E. Martínez, L. G. Baraldi, M. L. Louzada, et al., "Ultra-Processed Foods and Added Sugars in the US Diet: Evidence from a Nationally Representative Cross-Sectional Study," *BMJ Open*, 6 no. 3 (Mar 9, 2016): e009892, doi:10.1136/bmjopen-2015-009892.

132 A. E. Karpyn, D. Riser, T. Tracy, et al., "The Changing Landscape of Food Deserts," *UNSCN Nutr*, 44 (2019): 46–53, https://www.ncbi.nlm.nih.gov/pmc/articles/PMC7299236/.

Chapter 4: How to Eat an Elephant

133 B. M. Kuehn, "Heritage Diets and Culturally Appropriate Dietary Advice May Help Combat Chronic Disease," *JAMA*, 322 no. 23 (2019): 2271–2273, doi: 10.1001/jama.2019.18431.

134 Sara Baer-Sinnott, in discussion with the author, January 2020.

135 Sara Baer-Sinnott, in discussion with the author, January 2020.

136 E. Yoon, "The Grocery Industry Confronts a New Problem: Only 10 Percent of Americans Love Cooking," *Harvard Business Review*, September 22, 2017, accessed January 28, 2020, https://hbr.org/2017/09/the-grocery-industry-confronts-a-new-problem-only-10-of-americans-love-cooking.

137 S. Vedantam, "Creatures of Habit: How Habits Shape Who We Are—and Who We Become," NPR Hidden Brain, December 30, 2019, accessed October 8, 2021, https://www.npr.org/2019/12/11/787160734/creatures-of-habit-how-habits-shape-who-we-are-and-who-we-become.

Chapter 5: Dairy

138 "Lactose Intolerance: Diagnosis and Treatment," Mayo Clinic, accessed January 7, 2020, https://www.mayoclinic.org/diseases-conditions/lactose-intolerance/diagnosis-treatment/drc-20374238.

139 P. C. Kashyap, A. Marcobal, L. K. Ursell, et al., "Complex Interactions Among Diet, Gastrointestinal Transit, and Gut Microbiota in Humanized Mice," *Gastroenterology*, 144 no. 5 (2013): 967–977, doi:10.1053/j.gastro.2013.01.047.

140 L. Mulvany, "The Parmesan Cheese You Sprinkle on Your Penne Could Be Wood: Some Brands Promising 100 Percent Purity Contained No Parmesan at All," Bloomberg, February 16, 2016, accessed November 1, 2019, https://www.bloomberg.com/news/articles/2016-02-16/the-parmesan-cheese-you-sprinkle-on-your-penne-could-be-wood.

141 A. A. Dalhoff, S. B. Levy, "Does Use of the Polyene Natamycin as a Food Preservative Jeopardise the Clinical Efficacy of Amphotericin B? A Word of Concern," *Int J Antimicrob Agents*, 45 no. 6 (2015): 564–567, doi:10.1016/j.ijantimicag.2015.02.011.

142 G. B. Huffnagle, M. C. Noverr, "The Emerging World of the Fungal Microbiome," *Trends Microbiol*, 21 no. 7 (2013): 334–341, doi:10.1016/j.tim.2013.04.002.

143 C. E. Huseyin, P. W. O'Toole, P. D. Cotter, et al., "Forgotten Fungi—the Gut Mycobiome in Human Health and Disease, *FEMS Microbiol Rev*, 41 no. 4 (2017): 479–511, doi:10.1093/femsre/fuw047; L. Jiang, P. Stärkel, J. G. Fan, et al., "The Gut Mycobiome: A Novel Player in Chronic Liver Diseases," *J Gastroenterol*, 56 no. 1 (2021): 1–11, doi:10.1007/s00535-020-01740-5.

Chapter 6: Bread and Grains

144 P. Singh, A. Arora, T. A. Strand, et al., "Global Prevalence of Celiac Disease: Systematic Review and Meta-Analysis," *Clin Gastroenterol Hepatol*, 16 no. 6 (2018): 823–836.e2, doi:10.1016/j.cgh.2017.06.037.

145 J. R. Biesiekierski, E. D. Newnham, P. M. Irving, et al., "Gluten Causes Gastrointestinal Symptoms in Subjects Without Celiac Disease: A Double-Blind Randomized Placebo-Controlled Trial," *Am J Gastroenterol*, 106 no. 3 (Jan 11, 2011): 508.

146 M. I. Vazquez-Roque, M. Camilleri, T. Smyrk, et al., "A Controlled Trial of Gluten-Free Diet in Patients with Irritable Bowel Syndrome–Diarrhea: Effects on Bowel Frequency and Intestinal Function," *Gastroenterology*, 144 no. 5 (May 2013): 903–911.e3, doi: 10.1053/j.gastro.2013.01.049.

147 J. R. Biesiekierski, S. L. Peters, E. D. Newnham, et al., "No Effects of Gluten in Patients with Self-Reported Non-Celiac Gluten Sensitivity After Dietary Reduction of Fermentable, Poorly Absorbed, Short-Chain Carbohydrates," *Gastroenterology*, 145 no. 2 (Aug 2013): 320–8.e1-3, doi: 10.1053/j.gastro.2013.04.051.

148 J. Schwarcz, "Would Osler Stand by His Famous Quote Today?" McGill Office for Science and Society, March 20, 2017, accessed January 24, 2022, https://www.mcgill.ca/oss/article/controversial-science-health-history-news/would-osler-stand-his-famous-quote-today.

149 S. Naimi, et al., "Direct Impact," 2021.

150 E. Fee, T. M. Brown, "John Harvey Kellogg, MD: Health Reformer and Antismoking Crusader," *Am J Public Health*, 92 no. 6 (2002): 935, doi:10.2105/ajph.92.6.935.

151 M. Garber, "The Most Contentious," 2016.

152 A. Mayyasi, "Why Cereal Has Such Aggressive Marketing," *The Atlantic*, June 16, 2016, accessed August 31, 2020, https://www.theatlantic.com/business/archive/2016/06/how-marketers-invented-the-modern-version-of-breakfast/487130.

153 F. Laudisi, et al., "The Food Additive," 2019.

154 K. P. Nickerson, C. McDonald, "Crohn's Disease-Associated Adherent-Invasive *Escherichia coli* Adhesion Is Enhanced by Exposure to the Ubiquitous Dietary Polysaccharide Maltodextrin," *PloS ONE* 7 no.12 (Dec 12, 2012): e52132, doi:10.1371/journal.pone.0052132.

155 A. R. Arnold, B. Chassaing, "Maltodextrin, Modern Stressor of the Intestinal Environment," *Cell Mol Gastroenterol Hepatol*, 7 no. 2 (2019): 475–476, doi:10.1016/j.jcmgh.2018.09.014.

156 A. Brunning, "The Science of Making Porridge," Compound Interest, February 15, 2019, accessed August 27, 2020, https://www.compoundchem.com/2019/02/15/porridge/.

Chapter 7: Fruits and Vegetables

157 A. Fardet, E. Rock, "Perspective: Reductionist Nutrition Research Has Meaning Only Within the Framework of Holistic and Ethical Thinking," *Adv Nutr*, 9 no. 6 (2018): 655–670, doi:10.1093/advances/nmy044.

158 F. S. Atkinson , K. Foster-Powell, J. C. Brand-Miller, "International Tables of Glycemic Index and Glycemic Load Values: 2008," *Diabetes Care*, 31 no. 12 (2008): 2281–2283, doi:10.2337/dc08-1239.

159 A. Attaluri, R. Donahoe, J. Valestin, et al., "Randomised Clinical Trial: Dried Plums (Prunes) Vs. Psyllium for Constipation," *Aliment Pharmacol Ther*, 33 no. 7 (Apr 2011): 822–828, doi:10.1111/j.1365-2036.2011.04594.x.

160 B. A. Williams, D. Mikkelsen, B. M. Flanagan, et al., "Dietary Fibre": Moving Beyond the "Soluble/Insoluble" Classification for Monogastric Nutrition, with an Emphasis on Humans and Pigs," *J Animal Sci Biotechnol*, 10 no. 45 (2019), doi:10.1186/s40104-019-0350-9.

161 Zinöcker and Lindseth, "The Western Diet-," 2018

162 Zinöcker and Lindseth, "The Western Diet-," 2018.

163 B. Estabrook, Interview by I. Flatow, "The Unsavory Story of Industrially-Grown Tomatoes," *Talk of the Nation*, NPR, August 26, 2011, accessed October 28, 2019, https://www.npr.org/2011/08/26/139972669/the-unsavory-story-of-industrially-grown-tomatoes.

164 L. A. David, C. F. Maurice, R. N. Carmody, et al., "Diet Rapidly and Reproducibly Alters the Human Gut Microbiome," *Nature*, 505 no. 7484 (2014): 559–563, doi:10.1038/nature12820.

165 I. Lecklitner, "What's in This?: Tropicana Orange Juice," MEL Magazine, accessed August 28, 2020, https://melmagazine.com/en-us/story/whats-in-this-tropicana-orange-juice.

166 A. Bouzari, D. Holstege, D. M. Barrett, "Mineral, Fiber, and Total Phenolic Retention in Eight Fruits and Vegetables: A Comparison of Refrigerated and Frozen Storage," *J Agric Food Chem*, 63 no. 3 (2015): 951–956, doi:10.1021/jf504890k.

167 K. B. Comerford, "Frequent Canned Food Use Is Positively Associated with Nutrient-Dense Food Group Consumption and Higher Nutrient Intakes in US Children and Adults," *Nutrients*, 7 no. 7 (Jul 9, 2015): 5586–5600, doi:10.3390/nu7075240.

168 S. Jacoby, "Should You Try At-Home Food Sensitivity Tests?," Today Health and Wellness, January 25, 2022, accessed June 1, 2022, https://www.today.com/health/health/are-food-sensitivity-tests-accurate-rcna13271.

Chapter 8: Meat, Poultry, Eggs, and Other Proteins

169 E. Varian, "It's Called 'Plant Based,' Look It Up," *New York Times*, December 28, 2019, updated October 15, 2021, accessed March 23, 2022, https://www.nytimes.com/2019/12/28/style/plant-based-diet.html.

170 E. Varian, E, "It's Called 'Plant-Based,'" 2019.

171 A. Walansky, "Is Rotisserie Chicken Healthy? 5 Things to Look for at the Grocery Store," Today, May 17, 2019, accessed December 11, 2019, https://www.today.com/food/rotisserie-chicken-healthy-5-things-look-grocery-store-t154360.

172 J. Polivy, J. Coleman, C. P. Herman, "The Effect of Deprivation on Food Cravings and Eating Behavior in Restrained and Unrestrained Eaters," *Int J Eat Disord*, 38 no. 4 (2005): 301–309, doi:10.1002/eat.20195.

173 S. V. Irwin, P. Fisher, E. Graham, et al., "Sulfites Inhibit the Growth of Four Species of Beneficial Gut Bacteria at Concentrations Regarded as Safe for Food," *PLoS One*, 12 no. 10 (Oct 18, 2017): e0186629, doi:10.1371/journal.pone.0186629.

174 A. Levine, J.M. Rhodes, J.O. Lindsay, et al., "Dietary Guidance from the International Organization for the Study of Inflammatory Bowel Diseases," *Clin Gastroenterol Hepatol*, 18 no. 6 (2020): 1381–1392, doi:10.1016/j.cgh.2020.01.046

175 D. J. McNamara, "Dietary Cholesterol, Heart Disease Risk and Cognitive Dissonance," *Proc Nutr Soc*, 73 no. 2 (2014): 161–166, doi:10.1017/S0029665113003844.

176 C. Donat-Vargas, H. Sandoval-Insausti, J. Rey-García, et al., "High Consumption of Ultra-Processed Food Is Associated with Incident Dyslipidemia: A Prospective Study of Older Adults," *J Nutr*, 151 no. 8 (2021): 2390–2398, doi:10.1093/jn/nxab118.

177 F. Sofi, F. Cesari, R. Abbate, et al., "Adherence to Mediterranean Diet and Health Status: Meta-Analysis," *BMJ*, 337 (Sep 11, 2008): a1344, doi:10.1136/bmj.a1344.

Notes

Chapter 9: Desserts

178 M. Moss, *Hooked: Food, Free Will, and How the Food Giants Exploit Our Addictions* (New York: Random House, 2021), 49.

179 M. Moss, *Hooked*, 2021, 93.

180 M. J. Gibney, "Ultra-Processed Foods: Definitions and Policy Issues," *Curr Dev Nutr*, 3 no. 2 (Sep 14, 2018): nzy077, doi:10.1093/cdn/nzy077.

181 M. Pollan, *Cooked: A Natural History of Transformation* (New York: Penguin Press, 2013), 193.

182 M. Y. Park, "A History of the Cake Mix, the Invention that Redefined 'Baking,'" *Bon Appétit*, September 26, 2013, accessed December 10, 2019, https://www.bonappetit.com/entertaining-style/pop-culture/article/cake-mix-history.

Chapter 10: Drinks

183 M. D. Goncalves, C. Lu, J. Tutnauer, et al., "High-Fructose Corn Syrup Enhances Intestinal Tumor Growth in Mice," *Science*, 363 no. 6433 (2019): 1345–1349, doi:10.1126/science.aat8515.

184 J. J. DiNicolantonio, S. C. Lucan, "Is Fructose Malabsorption a Cause of Irritable Bowel Syndrome?," *Med Hypotheses*, 85 no. 3 (2015): 295–297, doi:10.1016/j.mehy.2015.05.019.

185 R. W. Walker, K. A. Dumke, M. I. Goran, "Fructose Content in Popular Beverages Made with and Without High-fructose Corn Syrup," *Nutrition*, 30 no. 7–8 (2014): 928–935, doi:10.1016/j.nut.2014.04.003.

186 "Distilled Spirits," US Food and Drug Administration, December 7, 2017, accessed March 25, 2022, https://www.fda.gov/about-fda/domestic-mous/distilled-spirits.

187 "The TTB Story," US Department of the Treasury, Alcohol and Tobacco Tax and Trade Bureau, updated February 14, 2018, accessed March 25, 2022, https://www.ttb.gov/about-ttb/history#:~:text=TTB%20was%20created%20in%20January,Treasury%2C%20and%20TTB%20was%20born.

188 "Determine If and How Ingredients May Be Used in Your Beverage," Alcohol and Tobacco Tax and Trade Bureau, updated December 3, 2018, accessed March 25, 2022, https://www.ttb.gov/formulation/determining-if-and-how-ingredients-may-be-used-in-your-beverage.

189 R. K. Bush, E. Zoratti, S. L. Taylor, "Diagnosis of Sulfite and Aspirin Sensitivity," *Clin Rev Allergy*, 8 no. 2–3 (1990):159–178, doi:10.1007/BF02914443.

190 C. W. Lecos, "Sulfites: FDA Limits Uses, Broadens Labeling [1986]," Food and Agriculture Organization of the United Nations, AGRIS, accessed March 25, 2022, https://agris.fao.org/agris-search/search.do?recordID=US8731341.

191 J. Stromberg J, "This Is Why Alcohol Doesn't Come with Nutrition Facts," Vox, updated March 14, 2015, accessed March 25, 2022, https://www.vox.com/2014/11/12/7195573/alcohol-nutrition.

192 "Food Additive Details: Gum Arabic (Acacia Gum)," GSFA Online, updated up to the 42nd Session of the Codex Alimentarius Commission (2019), accessed April 4, 2022, https://www.fao.org/gsfaonline/additives/details.html?id=63&d-3586470-s=5&lang=&d-3586470-o=2&print=true.

193 F. Bishehsari, E. Magno, G. Swanson, et al., "Alcohol and Gut-Derived Inflammation," *Alcohol Res*, 38 no. (2017): 163–171, https://www.ncbi.nlm.nih.gov/pmc/articles/PMC5513683/.

Chapter 11: Processed Foods

194 "Italians Try American Snacks," YouTube video, 2:31, posted by "BuzzFeedVideo, May 31, 2015, accessed November 29, 2019, https://www.youtube.com/watch?v=M1zuHZz9BXY.

195 K. P. Nickerson, R. Chanin, C. McDonald, "Deregulation of Intestinal Anti-Microbial Defense by the Dietary Additive, Maltodextrin," *Gut Microbes*, 6 no. 1 (2015): 78–83, doi:10.1080/19490976.2015.1005477.

196 "CFR—Code of Federal Regulations Title 21," US Food and Drug Administration, accessed November 30, 2019, https://www.accessdata.fda.gov/scripts/cdrh/cfdocs/cfcfr/CFRSearch.cfm?fr=172.836.

197 "Evaluation Report of Food Additives, Polysorbates (Polysorbate 20, Polysorbate 60, Polysorbate 65 and Polysorbate 80)," Japanese Food Safety Commission, June 2007, accessed November 30, 2019, https://www.fsc.go.jp/english/evaluationreports/foodadditive/polysorbate_report.pdf.

198 Japanese Food Safety Commission, "Evaluation Report of Food Additives," 2007.

199 C. L. Roberts, A. V. Keita, S. H. Duncan, et al., "Translocation of Crohn's Disease *Escherichia coli* across M-Cells: Contrasting Effects of Soluble Plant Fibres and Emulsifiers," *Gut*, 59 no. 10 (2010): 1331–1339, doi:10.1136/gut.2009.195370.

200 "Titanium Dioxide: E171 No Longer Considered Safe When Used as a Food Additive," EFSA—European Food Safety Authority, May 6, 2021, accessed November 29, 2021, https://www.efsa.europa.eu/en/news/titanium-dioxide-e171-no-longer-considered-safe-when-used-food-additive.

201 Levine, et al., "Dietary Guidance," 2020.

202 PubChem, "Glycerol (Compound)," NIH National Library of Medicine, accessed November 22, 2021, https://pubchem.ncbi.nlm.nih.gov/compound/753; Glycerin: Drug Information, UpToDate, accessed December 9, 2019, https://www.uptodate.com/contents/glycerin-drug-information?source=history_widget.

203 H. Markel, "The Secret Ingredient in Kellogg's Corn Flakes Is Seventh Day Adventism," *Smithsonian Magazine*, July 28, 2017, accessed November, 27, 2019, https://www.smithsonianmag.com/history/secret-ingredient-kelloggs-corn-flakes-seventh-day-adventism-180964247.

204 D. Gilliland, "Make Ketchup like Henry Heinz Used to Make," *Pittsburgh Post-Gazette*, October 13, 2017, accessed February 3, 2020, https://www.post-gazette.com/life/food/2017/10/13/Heinz-ketchup-octagon-bottle-keystone-recipe-pure-food/stories/201710160007.

205 Deborah Blum, *The Poison Squad* (New York: Penguin Press, 2018), 131–141.
206 Gilliland, "Make Ketchup," 2017.

Chapter 12: To Eat Out or Not to Eat Out?

207 M. J. Saksena, A. M. Okrent, T. D. Anekwe, et al., "America's Eating Habits: Food Away from Home," United States Department of Agriculture Economic Research Service, Economic Information Bulletin Number 196, September 2018, accessed December 20, 2021, https://www.ers.usda.gov/webdocs/publications/90228/eib-196.pdf?v=5683.8.

208 M. Pollan, "Cooked: A Natural History," 2013.

209 M. J. Saksena, et al., "America's Eating Habits," 2021.

210 "Table B-3: Average Hourly and Weekly Earnings of All Employees on Private Non-Farm Payrolls by Industry Sector, Seasonally Adjusted," US Bureau of Labor Statistics, Economic News Release, accessed December 23, 2019, www.bls.gov/news.release/empsit.t19.htm.

211 H. This, "Molecular Gastronomy, a Scientific Look at Cooking," *Acc Chem Res*, 42 no. 5 (May 19, 2009): 575–583, doi: 10.1021/ar8002078.

212 R. Burke, H. This, A. L. Kelly, "Molecular Gastronomy," Technological University Dublin, School of Culinary Arts and Food Technology, 2016, accessed December 20, 2021, https://arrow.tudublin.ie/cgi/viewcontent.cgi?article=1196&context=tfschafart.

213 "How to Cook with Agar Agar," Great British Chefs, accessed January 26, 2022, https://www.greatbritishchefs.com/how-to-cook/how-to-cook-with-agar-agar.

214 S. Naimi, et al., "Direct Impact," 2021.

215 S. Bertram, M. Kurland, E. Lydick, et al., "The Patient's Perspective of Irritable Bowel Syndrome," *J Fam Pract*, 50 no. 6 (Jun 2001): 521–525, https://pubmed.ncbi.nlm.nih.gov/11401739/.

Chapter 13: How to Eat Everything and Still Lose Weight

216 M. E. Lean, D. Malkova, "Altered Gut and Adipose Tissue Hormones in Overweight and Obese Individuals: Cause or Consequence?," *Int J Obes (Lond)*, 40 no. 4 (2016): 622–632, doi:10.1038/ijo.2015.220.

217 B. Chassaing, "Dietary Emulsifiers," 2015.

218 P. J. Turnbaugh, R. E. Ley, M. A. Mahowald, et al., "An Obesity-Associated Gut Microbiome with Increased Capacity for Energy Harvest," *Nature*, 444 no. 7122 (2006): 1027–1031, doi:10.1038/nature05414.

219 M. G. Novelle, "Decoding the Role of Gut-Microbiome in the Food Addiction Paradigm," *Int J Environ Res Public Health*, 18 no. 13 (Jun 25, 2021): 6825, doi:10.3390/ijerph18136825.

220 K. D. Hall, A. Ayuketah, R. Brychta, et al., "Ultra-Processed Diets Cause Excess Calorie Intake and Weight Gain: An Inpatient Randomized Controlled Trial of Ad Libitum Food Intake," *Cell Metab*, 30 no. 1 (Jul 2, 2019): 67–77.e3, doi: 10.1016/j.cmet.2019.05.008.

221 A. A. Kolodziejczyk, D. Zheng, E. Elinav, "Diet-Microbiota Interactions and Personalized Nutrition," *Nat Rev Microbiol*, 17 no. 12 (2019): 742–753, doi:10.1038/s41579-019-0256-8.

222 K. D. Hall, J. Guo, A. B. Courville, et al., "Effect of a Plant-Based, Low-Fat Diet Versus an Animal-Based, Ketogenic Diet on Ad Libitum Energy Intake," *Nat Med*, 27 no. 2 (2021): 344–353, doi:10.1038/s41591-020-01209-1.

223 A. Żarrinpar, A. Chaix, S. Yooseph S, et al., "Diet and Feeding Pattern Affect the Diurnal Dynamics of the Gut Microbiome," *Cell Metab*, 20 no. 6 (2014): 1006–1017, doi:10.1016/j.cmet.2014.11.008.

224 T. M. Halliday, M. H. White, A. K. Hild, et al., "Appetite and Energy Intake Regulation in Response to Acute Exercise," *Med Sci Sports Exerc*, 53 no. 10102021): 2173–2181, doi:10.1249/MSS.0000000000002678.

Chapter 14: Troubleshooting

225 E. Ma, G. Maskarinec, U. Lim, et al., "Long-Term Association Between Diet Quality and Characteristics of the Gut Microbiome in the Multiethnic Cohort Study, *Br J Nutr*, 2021: 1–10, doi:10.1017/S0007114521002968.

226 Wastyk, et al., "Gut-Microbiota-Targeted Diets," 2021.

227 J. G. Mills, P. Weinstein, N. J. C. Gellie, et al., "Urban Habitat Restoration Provides a Human Health Benefit Through Microbiome Rewilding: The Microbiome Rewilding Hypothesis," *Restor Ecol*, 25 (2017): 866–872, doi:10.1111/rec.12610.

228 M. D. Brown, L. M. Shinn, G. Reeser, et al., "Fecal and Soil Microbiota Composition of Gardening and Non-Gardening Families," *Sci Rep*, 12 no. 1 (Jan 31, 2022): 1595, doi:10.1038/s41598-022-05387-5.

229 D. Kviatcovsky, D. Zheng, E. Elinav, "Gut Microbiome and Its Potential Link to Personalized Nutrition," *Science Direct Current Opinion in Physiology*, 22 (2021): 100439,https://doi.org/10.1016/j.cophys.2021.05.002.

230 U.S. National Library of Medicine, "Predict 2: Personalized Responses to Dietary Composition Trial 2," accessed April 4, 2022, https://clinicaltrials.gov/ct2/show/NCT03983733.

231 M. El-Salhy, J. G. Hatlebakk, O. H. Gilja, et al., "Efficacy of Faecal Microbiota Transplantation for Patients with Irritable Bowel Syndrome in a Randomised, Double-Blind, Placebo-Controlled Study," *Gut*, 69 (2020): 859–867, doi: 10.1136/gutjnl-2019-319630.

232 K. Servick, "Pill Derived from Human Feces Treats Recurrent Gut Infections," *Science*, January 19, 2022, accessed April 4, 2022, https://www.science.org/content/article/pill-derived-human-feces-treats-recurrent-gut-infections.

233 A. Iriondo-DeHond, J. A. Uranga, M. D. Del Castillo, et al., "Effects of Coffee and Its Components on the Gastrointestinal Tract and the Brain-Gut Axis," *Nutrients*, 13 no. 1 (Dec 29, 2020): 88, doi:10.3390/nu13010088.

234 M. T. Bernstein, L. A. Graff, L. Avery, et al., "Gastrointestinal Symptoms Before and During Menses in Healthy Women," *BMC Womens Health*, 14 (Jan 22, 2014): 14, doi:10.1186/1472-6874-14-14.

235 S. V. Kane, K. Sable, S. B. Hanauer, "The Menstrual Cycle and Its Effect on Inflammatory Bowel Disease and Irritable Bowel Syndrome: A Prevalence Study," *Am J Gastroenterol*, 93 no. 10 (1998): 1867–1872, doi:10.1111/j.1572-0241.1998.540_i.x.

236 A. M. Case, R. L. Reid, "Effects of the Menstrual Cycle on Medical Disorders," *Arch Intern Med*, 158 no. 13 (1998): 1405–1412, doi:10.1001/archinte.158.13.1405.

237 M. Trottier, A. Erebara, P. Bozzo, "Treating Constipation During Pregnancy," *Can Fam Physician*, 58 no. 8 (2012): 836–838, https://www.ncbi.nlm.nih.gov/pmc/articles/PMC3418980/.

Conclusion: Cooking up Change

238 "Packaged Food Market," Market Research Future, April 2021, accessed September 22, 2021, https://www.marketresearchfuture.com/reports/packaged-food-market-10540.

239 B. Srour, L. K. Fezeu, E. Kesse-Guyot, et al., "Ultra-Processed Food Intake and Risk of Cardiovascular Disease: Prospective Cohort Study (NutriNet-Santé)," *BMJ*, 365 (May 29, 2019): l1451, doi:10.1136/bmj.l1451.

240 E. Reed, "The Average Cost of Food in America," The Street Smarts, January 25, 2019, updated April 3, 2020, accessed June 5, 2022, https://www.thestreet.com/personal-finance/average-cost-of-food-14845479.

241 L. Garfield, "American Fast Food as We Know It Is Dying—and Healthier Chains May Be Replacing It," Business Insider, November 15, 2017, accessed January 26, 2022, https://www.businessinsider.com/future-of-fast-food-healthy-affordable-2017-11.

Appendix A: Additives to Avoid (and Why)

242 Lichtenstein, et al., "2021 Dietary Guidance," 2021.

243 Levine, et al., "Dietary Guidance," 2020.

244 Ministry of Health of Brazil, "Dietary Guidelines," 2015.

245 "Food-Based Dietary Guidelines—Uruguay," Food and Agriculture Organization of the United Nations, 2016, accessed January 3, 2022, https://www.fao.org/nutrition/education/food-dietary-guidelines/regions/uruguay/en/.

246 S. F. Bhat, S. E. Pinney, K. M. Kennedy, et al., "Exposure to High Fructose Corn Syrup During Adolescence in the Mouse Alters Hepatic Metabolism and the Microbiome in a Sex-Specific Manner," *J Physiol*, 599 no. 5 (2021): 1487–1511, doi:10.1113/JP280034.

247 Y. Lebenthal-Bendor, R. C. Theuer, A. Lebenthal, et al., "Malabsorption of Modified Food Starch (Acetylated Distarch Phosphate) in Normal Infants and in 8-24-Month-Old Toddlers

with Non-Specific Diarrhea, as Influenced by Sorbitol and Fructose," *Acta Paediatr*, 90 no. 12 (2001): 1368–1372, doi:10.1080/08035250152708734.

248 M. I. Goran, S. J. Ulijaszek, E. E. Ventura, "High Fructose Corn Syrup and Diabetes Prevalence: A Global Perspective," *Glob Public Health*, 8 no. 1 (2013): 55–64, doi:10.1080/174416 92.2012.736257.

249 K. L. Stanhope, A. A. Bremer, V. Medici, et al., "Consumption of Fructose and High Fructose Corn Syrup Increase Postprandial Triglycerides, LDL-Cholesterol, and Apolipoprotein-B in Young Men and Women," *J Clin Endocrinol Metab*, 96 no. 10 (2011): E1596–E1605, doi: 10.1210/jc.2011-1251.

250 J. Todoric, G. Di Caro, S. Reibe, et al., "Fructose Stimulated De Novo Lipogenesis Is Promoted by Inflammation," *Nat Metab*, 2 no. 10 (2020): 1034–1045, doi:10.1038/s42255-020-0261-2.

251 M. D. Goncalves, C. Lu, J. Tutnauer, et al., "High-Fructose Corn Syrup Enhances Intestinal Tumor Growth in Mice," *Science*, 363 no. 6433 (2019): 1345–1349, doi:10.1126/science. aat8515.

252 EFSA Panel on Food Additives and Flavourings (FAF), M. Younes, G. Aquilina, et al., "Safety of a Proposed Amendment of the Specifications for Steviol Glycosides (E 960) as a Food Additive: to Expand the List of Steviol Glycosides to All Those Identified in the Leaves of *Stevia Rebaudiana Bertoni*," *EFSA Journal. European Food Safety Authority*, no. 18 (4) (2020): e06106, doi:10.2903/j.efsa.2020.6106.

253 A. Callahan, "Are There Downsides to the Sweetener Stevia?" *New York Times*, May 4, 2018, accessed January 3, 2022, https://www.nytimes.com/2018/05/04/well/eat/stevia-sweetener-sugar-side-effects-downsides.html.

254 X. Bian, L. Chi, B. Gao, et al., "Gut Microbiome Response to Sucralose and Its Potential Role in Inducing Liver Inflammation in Mice," *Front Physiol*, 8 (Jul 24, 2017): 487, doi: 10.3389/fphys.2017.00487.

255 Bian, et al., "Gut Microbiome Response," 2017.

256 J. Slavin, "Fiber and Prebiotics: Mechanisms and Health Benefits," *Nutrients*, 5 no. 4 (Apr 22, 2013): 1417–1435, doi:10.3390/nu5041417.

257 Zinöcker and Lindseth, "The Western Diet," 2018.

258 C. Holland, P. Ryden, C. H. Edwards, et al., "Plant Cell Walls: Impact on Nutrient Bioaccessibility and Digestibility," *Foods*, 9 no. 2 (Feb 16, 2020): 201, doi:10.3390/foods9020201.

259 S. Naimi, et al., "Direct Impact," 2021.

260 M. F. de Jesus Raposo, A. M. de Morais, R. M. de Morai, "Emergent Sources of Prebiotics: Seaweeds and Microalgae," *Mar Drugs*, 14 no. 2 (Jan 28, 2016): 27, doi:10.3390/md14020027.

261 J. V. Martino, et al., "The Role of Carrageenan," 2017.

262 B. Borsani, R. De Santis, V. Perico, et al., "The Role of Carrageenan in Inflammatory Bowel Diseases and Allergic Reactions: Where Do We Stand?" *Nutrients*, 13 no. 10 (Sep 27, 2021): 3402, doi:10.3390/nu13103402.

263 C. Chassard, E. Delmas, C. Robert, et al., "The Cellulose-Degrading Microbial Community of the Human Gut Varies According to the Presence or Absence of Methanogens," *FEMS Microbiology Ecology*, 74 no. 1 (Oct 1, 2010;): 205–213, doi:10.1111/j.1574-6941.2010.00941.x.

Notes

264 Z. Liu, H. Liu, A. M. Vera, et al., "High Force Catch Bond Mechanism of Bacterial Adhesion in the Human Gut," *Nat Commun*, 11 no. 1 (Aug 28, 2020): 4321, doi:10.1038/s41467-020-18063-x.

265 S. Naimi, "Direct Impact," 2021.

266 A. Mortensen, F. Aguilar, R. Crebelli, et al., "Re-Evaluation of Acacia Gum (E 414) as a Food Additive," *EFSA J*, 15 no. 4 (2017): e04741, doi:10.2903/j.efsa.2017.4741.

267 J. Juśkiewicz, Z. Zduńczyk, "Effects of Cellulose, Carboxymethylcellulose and Inulin Fed to Rats as Single Supplements or in Combinations on Their Caecal Parameters," *Comp Biochem Physiol A Mol Integr Physiol*, 139 no. 4 (Dec 2004): 513–519, PMID: 15596397.

268 J. V. Martino, et al., "The Role of Carrageenan," 2017.

269 "Gellan Gum," IPCS INCHEM Summary of Evaluations Performed by the Joint FAO/WHO Expert Committee on Food Additives, accessed January 5, 2022, https://inchem.org/documents/jecfa/jeceval/jec_896.htm.

270 P. A. Todd, P. Benfield , K. L. Goa, "Guar Gum, A Review of Its Pharmacological Properties, and Use as a Dietary Adjunct in Hypercholesterolaemia," *Drugs*, 39 no. 6 (Jun 1990): 917–928, doi:10.2165/00003495-199039060-00007.

271 A. Mortensen, F. Aguilar, R. Crebelliet, et al., "Re-Evaluation of Locust Bean Gum (E 410) as a Food Additive," *EFSA J*, 15 no. 1 (Jan 20, 2017): e04646, doi:10.2903/j.efsa.2017.4646.

272 J. Daly, J. Tomlin, N. W. Read, "The Effect of Feeding Xanthan Gum on Colonic Function in Man: Correlation with in Vitro Determinants of Bacterial Breakdown," *Br J Nutr*, 69 no. 3 (May 1993): 897–902, doi: 10.1079/bjn19930089.

273 C. A. Edwards, M. A. Eastwood, "Caecal and Faecal Short-Chain Fatty Acids and Stool Output in Rats Fed on Diets Containing Non-Starch Polysaccharides," *Br J Nutr*, 73 no. 5 (May 1995): 773–81, doi: 10.1079/bjn19950080.

274 M. A. Eastwood, W. G. Brydon, D. M. Anderson, "The Dietary Effects of Xanthan Gum in Man," *Food Addit Contam*, 4 no. 1 (Jan-Mar 1987): 17–26, doi: 10.1080/02652038709373610.

275 D. Vandeputte, G. Falony, S. Vieira-Silva, et al., "Prebiotic Inulin-Type Fructans Induce Specific Changes in the Human Gut Microbiota," *Gut*, 66 no. 11 (2017): 1968–1974, doi:10.1136/gutjnl-2016-313271.

276 V. Singh, B. S. Yeoh, B. Chassaing, et al., "Dysregulated Microbial Fermentation of Soluble Fiber Induces Cholestatic Liver Cancer," *Cell*, 175 no. 3 (2018): 679–694.e22, doi:10.1016/j.cell.2018.09.004.

277 Y. Lebenthal-Bendor, et al., "Malabsorption of Modified Food Starch," 2001.

278 National Collaborating Centre for Nursing and Supportive Care (UK), "Irritable Bowel Syndrome in Adults: Diagnosis and Management of Irritable Bowel Syndrome in Primary Care [Internet]," London: Royal College of Nursing (UK), Feb 2008, https://www.ncbi.nlm.nih.gov/books/NBK51960/.

279 K. P. Nickerson, C. McDonald, "Crohn's Disease–Associated Adherent-Invasive *Escherichia coli* Adhesion Is Enhanced by Exposure to the Ubiquitous Dietary Polysaccharide Maltodextrin," *PloS One*, 7 no. 12 (2012): e52132, doi:10.1371/journal.pone.0052132.

280 K. P. Nickerson, "Crohn's Disease–Associated Adherent-Invasive *Escherichia coli*" 2012.

281 S. Naimi, "Direct Impact," 2021.

Notes

282 H. Song, W. Chai, F. Yang, et al., "Effects of Dietary Monoglyceride and Diglyceride Supplementation on the Performance, Milk Composition, and Immune Status of Sows During Late Gestation and Lactation," *Front Vet Sci*, 8 (Aug 16, 2021): 714068, doi:10.3389/fvets.2021.714068.

283 R. G. Nejrup, T. R. Licht, L. I. Hellgren, "Fatty Acid Composition and Phospholipid Types Used in Infant Formulas Modifies the Establishment of Human Gut Bacteria in Germ-Free Mice," *Sci Rep*, 7 no. 1 (Jun 21, 2017): 3975, doi:10.1038/s41598-017-04298-0.

284 "Lecithin," University of Rochester Medical Center Health Encyclopedia, accessed December 4, 2019, https://www.urmc.rochester.edu/encyclopedia/content.aspx?contenttypeid=19&contentid=Lecithin.

285 B. Chassaing, T. Van de Wiele, J. De Bodt J, et al., "Dietary Emulsifiers Directly Alter Human Microbiota Composition and Gene Expression Ex Vivo Potentiating Intestinal Inflammation," *Gut*, 66 no. 8 (2017): 1414–1427, doi:10.1136/gutjnl-2016-313099.

286 E. Viennois, D. Merlin, A. T. Gewirtz, et al., "Dietary Emulsifier–Induced Low-Grade Inflammation Promotes Colon Carcinogenesis," *Cancer Res.*, 77 no. 1 (2017): 27–40, doi:10.1158/0008-5472.CAN-16-1359.

287 R. De Weirdt, S. Possemiers, G. Vermeulen, et al., "Human Faecal Microbiota Display Variable Patterns of Glycerol Metabolism," *FEMS Microbiol Ecol*, 74 no. 3 (2010): 601–611, doi:10.1111/j.1574-6941.2010.00974.x

288 A. Mortensen, F. Aguilar, R. Crebelliet, et al., "Re-Evaluation of Glycerol (E 422) as a Food Additive," *EFSA J*, 15 no. 3 Mar 15, 2017): e04720, doi:10.2903/j.efsa.2017.4720.

289 A. Lenhart, et al., "A Systematic Review," 2017.

290 A. Lenhart, et al., "A Systematic Review," 2017.

291 J. Däbritz, M. Mühlbauer, D. Domagk, et al., "Significance of Hydrogen Breath Tests in Children with Suspected Carbohydrate Malabsorption," *BMC Pediatr*, 14 (Feb 27, 2014): 59, doi:10.1186/1471-2431-14-59.

292 A. Lenhart, et al., "A Systematic Review," 2017.

293 P. A. Ruiz, B. Morón , H. M. Becker, et al., "Titanium Dioxide Nanoparticles Exacerbate DSS-Induced Colitis: Role of the NLRP3 Inflammasome," *Gut*, 66 no. 7 (2017): 1216–1224, doi:10.1136/gutjnl-2015-310297.

294 A. Levine, J. M. Rhodes, J. O. Lindsay, et al., "Dietary Guidance from the International Organization for the Study of Inflammatory Bowel Diseases," *Clin Gastroenterol Hepatol*, 18 no. 6 (2020): 1381–1392, doi:10.1016/j.cgh.2020.01.046.

295 "Titanium Dioxide: E171 No Longer Considered Safe When Used as a Food Additive," EFSA—European Food Safety Authority, May 6, 2021, accessed November 29, 2021, https://www.efsa.europa.eu/en/news/titanium-dioxide-e171-no-longer-considered-safe-when-used-food-additive.

Index

Index

Index

Index

O

oatmeal, 93–94, 155
obesity, 14
Oldways, 66–67
Olendzki, Barbara, 49, 65, 170
oligosaccharides, 24–25
Olive Oil Cake, 232–233
organic products, 47, 82
Osler, William, 88
Oven "Fried" Chicken, 212–214

P

pain medication, 176
Paleo diet, 152
Palm Beach, Fla., 51–52
pancakes, 94–95
partially hydrogenated oils, 58
pastas, 90–91, 153
pasteurization, 83
Perfect Breakfast Granola, 207–208
perfectionism, 70–71
pizza restaurants, 152
plant-based diets, 109–111, 173–174, 209
The Poison Squad (Blum), 40
Pollan, Michael, 120, 161
polyols, 16, 125, 194–195
polysaccharides, 188–189
polysorbate 60, 119, 120, 134, 194
polysorbate 80, 47, 119, 134, 194
prebiotic foods, 49, 55–57
prebiotics, 45, 46, 105, 159
prediabetes, 15–17, 127
PREDICT studies, 171–172
premade iced teas, 126–127
premixed spices, 137–138
preservatives, 79, 113, 128, 158
probiotic foods, 49, 56–57, 129, 170
probiotic supplements, 56–57, 170
processed foods, 6, 131–140
    in making less processed meals, 136–140
    meats, 112–114

in Nova classification system, 35, 36
and risk of cancer, 23
snack foods, 133–135
technologies for, 34–35
throughout history, 34
ultra-processed foods vs., 132 (*see also* ultra-processed foods)
progesterone, 177
prostaglandins, 177
proteins, 109–116
    body's processing of, 160–161
    with breakfast, 107
    chicken, 111–112
    eggs, 97, 115–116
    processed meats, 112–114
    shrimp and seafood, 114–115
    vegetarian, 110–111
psyllium, 99–100
public health issue, ultra-processed food as, 52–53, 62–63
Pure Food and Drug Act of 1906, 139

R

real food. *see also* whole foods
    cooking (*see* cooking at home)
    cost of, 181–182
    difficulty in finding/eating, 65–72
    eating like your ancestors, 66–68
    effect of food additives vs., 28
    recipes for (*see* recipes)
    transitioning from ultra-processed food to, 65–66
    transitioning to, 69–72
    and weight, 157–159, 162
Real Hot Cocoa, 233–234
Really Easy Homemade Whipped Cream, 234–235
recipes, 201–235. *see also individual categories of recipes*
    for ancestral dishes, 68–69
    bread and bread alternatives, 201–206

270

Index

About the Author

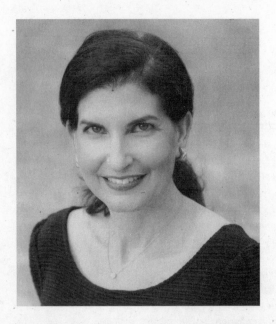

Dr. Dawn Harris Sherling is a board-certified internal medicine physician. She began studying journalism before switching to pre-med studies at the University of Florida. She earned her MD from the Yale University School of Medicine and then completed her residency at Harvard's Brigham and Women's Hospital where she went on to serve as an attending physician and also was Instructor in Medicine at Harvard University. She moved back to her native Florida, where she currently sees patients at a clinic for underserved populations and is an associate program director for the internal medicine residency at the Charles E. Schmidt College of Medicine at Florida Atlantic University.